Welcome to the ***"Anti-Inflammatory 5-Ingredient Cookbook: 5-Ingredient Recipes to Naturally Reduce Inflammation and Enhance Wellness."*** This cookbook is designed to make healthy eating easy, accessible, and enjoyable by focusing on recipes that require only five simple ingredients. Our goal is to help you harness the power of anti-inflammatory foods to support your health and well-being.

Why This Cookbook?

In today's fast-paced world, it can be challenging to find time to prepare nutritious meals. This cookbook simplifies the process by providing you with delicious and effective anti-inflammatory recipes that are quick and easy to make. Whether you're new to cooking or a seasoned chef, you'll find these recipes straightforward and satisfying.

What You'll Discover Inside:

- ***Simple and Delicious Recipes:*** Enjoy over 100 recipes that focus on reducing inflammation using just five key ingredients. From breakfasts and main dishes to snacks and desserts, each recipe is crafted to maximize flavor and health benefits with minimal effort.

- ***Health Benefits:*** Learn about the powerful anti-inflammatory properties of various ingredients and how they can help reduce inflammation, alleviate pain, and improve overall wellness.

- ***Easy-to-Follow Instructions:*** Each recipe is designed to be simple and clear, making it easy for anyone to follow along and create nutritious meals.

- ***Practical Tips:*** Gain valuable insights into meal planning, grocery shopping, and ingredient substitutions to make anti-inflammatory cooking a seamless part of your daily routine.

Why Choose Anti-Inflammatory Foods?

- ***Reduced Pain and Discomfort:*** Anti-inflammatory foods can help decrease chronic inflammation, which is often associated with conditions such as arthritis, heart disease, and diabetes.

- ***Improved Overall Health:*** Incorporating these foods into your diet can lead to better digestion, increased energy levels, and enhanced immune function.

- ***Natural Healing:*** By focusing on whole, unprocessed ingredients, you can support your body's natural healing processes and promote long-term wellness.

Whether you're looking to manage a specific health condition or simply want to improve your overall diet, the "Anti-Inflammatory 5-Ingredient Cookbook" is here to guide you. Embrace the simplicity and power of five-ingredient recipes to naturally reduce inflammation and enhance your wellness. With this cookbook, you'll discover that eating healthily doesn't have to be complicated or time-consuming—it can be easy, delicious, and incredibly rewarding.

Let's embark on this journey to better health and vitality together!

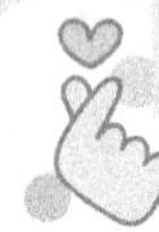

Procedure:

1. Preheat grill to medium•high heat.

2. Brush the salmon fillets with olive oil and season with salt and pepper.

3. Grill the salmon for 4•6 minutes per side, or until it flakes easily with a fork.

4. Squeeze fresh lemon juice over the grilled salmon.

5. Sprinkle with chopped fresh dill.

The key anti•inflammatory ingredients in this recipe are:

1. Salmon • Rich in omega•3 fatty acids, which have potent anti•inflammatory properties.

2. Lemon • Contains vitamin C and citric acid, which can help reduce inflammation.

3. Olive oil • Contains monounsaturated fats and polyphenols that have anti•inflammatory effects.

4. Dill • Contains flavonoids and other compounds with anti•inflammatory benefits.

This simple, 5•ingredient grilled salmon dish is a great option for an easy, healthy, and anti•inflammatory meal.

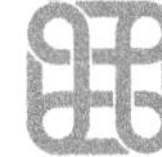

What is the total cooking time, including prep time?

Prep Time : ______________

Cook Time : ______________

Servings   : ______________

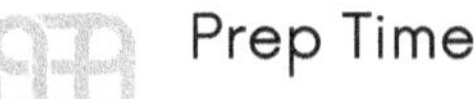 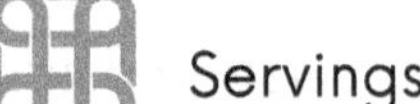

Ingredients:

 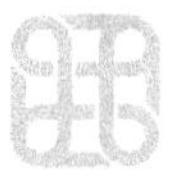

1. Salmon fillets
2. Lemon juice
3. Olive oil
4. Fresh dill
5. Salt and pepper

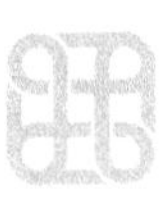 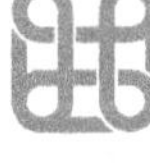 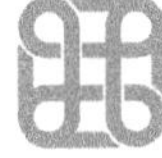 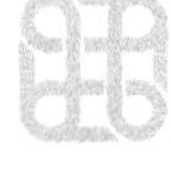 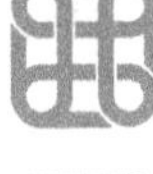 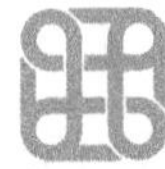

Is the recipe easy to follow?

1. Grilled salmon with lemon and dill

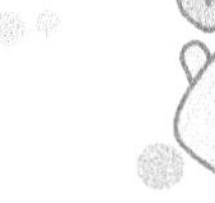

What are the critical points in the recipe (e.g., temperature control, timing)?

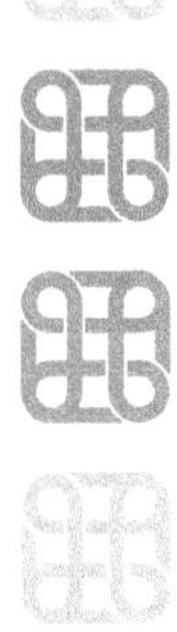

What is the total cooking time, including prep time?

Prep Time : ___________________

Cook Time : ___________________

Servings : ___________________

Ingredients:

- 1 head of cauliflower, cut into florets
- 2 tablespoons olive oil
- 1 teaspoon ground turmeric
- 1/2 teaspoon salt
- 1/4 teaspoon black pepper

Is the recipe easy to follow?

2. Turmeric roasted cauliflower

1. Preheat your oven to 400°F (200°C).

2. In a large bowl, toss the cauliflower florets with the olive oil, turmeric, salt, and black pepper until the cauliflower is evenly coated.

3. Spread the seasoned cauliflower florets in a single layer on a baking sheet.

4. Roast in the preheated oven for 20·25 minutes, or until the cauliflower is tender and lightly browned on the edges.

5. Serve the turmeric roasted cauliflower warm, as a side dish or snack.

That's it! This simple 5·ingredient recipe allows the natural sweetness of the cauliflower to shine, while the turmeric adds a beautiful golden color and earthy flavor.

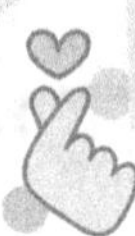

What are the critical points in the recipe (e.g., temperature control, timing)?

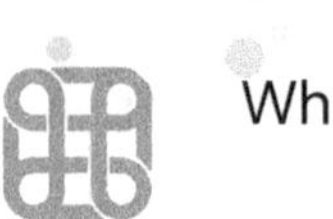

What is the total cooking time, including prep time?

Prep Time : ________________

Cook Time : ________________

Servings : ________________

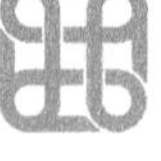

Ingredients:

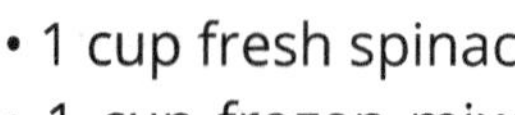

• 1 cup fresh spinach
• 1 cup frozen mixed berries (such as blueberries, raspberries, and strawberries)
• 1 cup unsweetened almond milk
• 1 tablespoon honey (or maple syrup for a vegan option)
• 1 tablespoon ground flaxseed

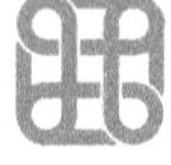
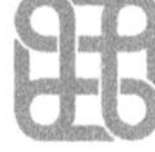
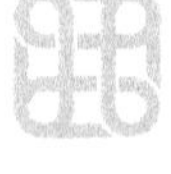
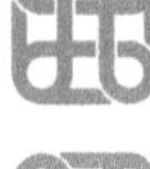
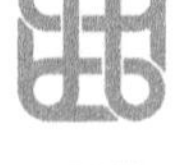

Is the recipe easy to follow?

3. Spinach and berry smoothie

1. Add the spinach, frozen berries, almond milk, honey (or maple syrup), and ground flaxseed to a high•speed blender.

2. Blend on high speed until the mixture is smooth and creamy, about 1•2 minutes.

3. Pour the smoothie into a glass and enjoy immediately.

This smoothie is packed with anti•inflammatory ingredients:

• Spinach is a nutrient•dense leafy green that is rich in antioxidants and anti•inflammatory compounds.
• Berries are high in antioxidants and have been shown to have potent anti•inflammatory properties.
• Flaxseed is a great source of anti•inflammatory omega•3 fatty acids.
• Almond milk is a dairy•free, low•calorie option that is also anti•inflammatory.
• Honey (or maple syrup) provides a natural sweetener without the inflammatory effects of refined sugar.

This smoothie is a delicious and healthy way to support an anti•inflammatory diet. Enjoy it as a nutritious breakfast or snack.

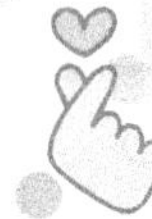

What are the critical points in the recipe (e.g., temperature control, timing)?

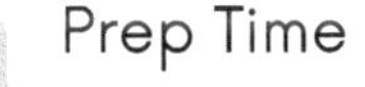

What is the total cooking time, including prep time?

Prep Time : ______________________

Cook Time : ______________________

Servings : ______________________

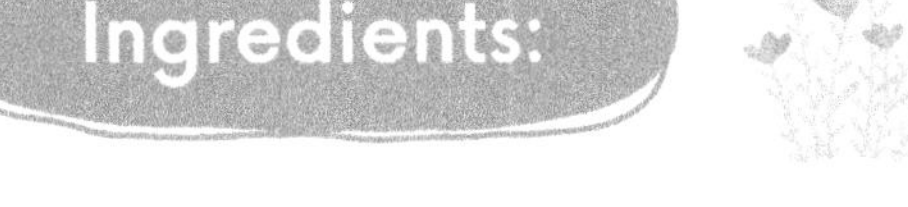
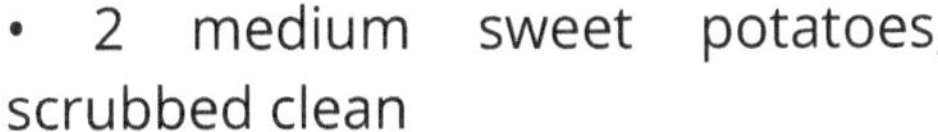

Ingredients:

- 2 medium sweet potatoes, scrubbed clean
- 1 tablespoon olive oil
- 1 teaspoon ground cinnamon
- 1/4 teaspoon ground ginger (optional)
- 1/4 teaspoon sea salt

Is the recipe easy to follow?

4. Baked sweet potato with cinnamon

1. Preheat your oven to 400°F (200°C).

2. Pierce the sweet potatoes several times with a fork. This will allow steam to escape during baking.

3. Rub the sweet potatoes all over with the olive oil.

4. In a small bowl, mix together the cinnamon, ginger (if using), and sea salt.

5. Sprinkle the cinnamon•spice mixture evenly over the oiled sweet potatoes, rubbing it in gently to coat them.

6. Place the seasoned sweet potatoes directly on the oven rack and bake for 45•60 minutes, or until they are very soft when pierced with a fork.

7. Remove the baked sweet potatoes from the oven and let them cool for 5 minutes.

8. Slice the sweet potatoes open and serve warm, with any juices spooned over the top.

This simple baked sweet potato dish is an excellent anti•inflammatory option:

- Sweet potatoes are rich in beta•carotene, an antioxidant with potent anti•inflammatory properties.
- Cinnamon has been shown to have strong anti•inflammatory effects.
- Ginger is another powerful anti•inflammatory spice.
- Olive oil provides healthy fats that can help reduce inflammation.

Enjoy this comforting and nutritious baked sweet potato as a side dish or a satisfying snack.

What is the total cooking time, including prep time?

Prep Time   : _______________

Cook Time : _______________

Servings   : _______________

Ingredients:

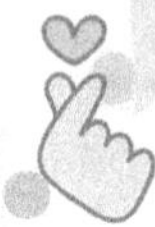

• 2 slices of whole•grain or sourdough bread
• 1 ripe avocado, mashed
• 1 tablespoon extra•virgin olive oil
• 1/4 teaspoon sea salt
• 1/4 teaspoon ground black pepper

Is the recipe easy to follow?

5. Avocado toast with olive oil

Procedure:

1. Toast the bread slices until lightly golden brown.

2. In a small bowl, mash the avocado with a fork until it reaches your desired consistency.

3. Drizzle the extra•virgin olive oil over the mashed avocado and mix well to combine.

4. Season the avocado mixture with sea salt and ground black pepper, and stir to incorporate.

5. Spread the seasoned avocado mixture evenly over the toasted bread slices.

6. Serve the avocado toast immediately, while the bread is still warm.

This simple avocado toast is an excellent anti•inflammatory option:

• Avocado is a rich source of healthy monounsaturated fats, which have been shown to have anti•inflammatory properties.
• Olive oil is also high in anti•inflammatory monounsaturated fats, as well as antioxidants.
• Whole•grain or sourdough bread provides complex carbohydrates and fiber, which can help reduce inflammation.
• Sea salt and black pepper are both natural anti•inflammatory seasonings.

This avocado toast makes for a nutritious and satisfying breakfast or snack that supports an anti•inflammatory diet. Enjoy it as a quick and easy way to incorporate more anti•inflammatory foods into your daily routine.

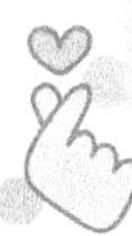

Procedure:

What is the total cooking time, including prep time?

Prep Time : ___________________

Cook Time : ___________________

Servings : ___________________

Ingredients:

- 1/4 cup chia seeds
- 1 cup unsweetened almond milk
- 1 tablespoon honey (or maple syrup for a vegan option)
- 1 cup mixed berries (such as blueberries, raspberries, and strawberries)
- 1/4 teaspoon ground cinnamon

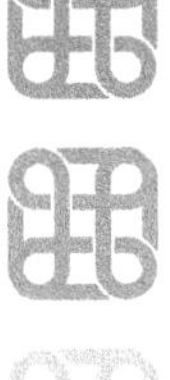
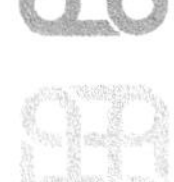
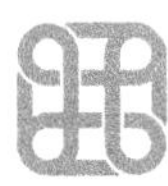
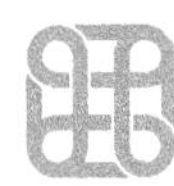

Is the recipe easy to follow?

6. *Chia seed pudding with berries*

1. In a medium•sized bowl, whisk together the chia seeds and almond milk until well combined.

2. Stir in the honey (or maple syrup) and mix until dissolved.

3. Cover the bowl and refrigerate the chia seed pudding for at least 2 hours, or overnight, stirring occasionally, until it has thickened to a pudding•like consistency.

4. When ready to serve, divide the chia seed pudding into serving bowls or glasses.

5. Top each portion with the mixed berries and a sprinkle of ground cinnamon.

This chia seed pudding is an excellent anti•inflammatory option:

- Chia seeds are a great source of anti•inflammatory omega•3 fatty acids.
- Berries are high in antioxidants and have been shown to have potent anti•inflammatory properties.
- Almond milk is a dairy•free, low•calorie option that is also anti•inflammatory.
- Honey (or maple syrup) provides a natural sweetener without the inflammatory effects of refined sugar.
- Cinnamon is a spice with strong anti•inflammatory benefits.

This chia seed pudding makes for a delicious and nutritious breakfast or snack that supports an anti•inflammatory diet. Enjoy it chilled and topped with the fresh, vibrant berries.

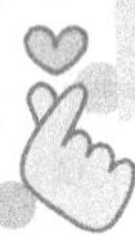

Procedure:

What is the total cooking time,
including prep time?

Prep Time : _______________

Cook Time : _______________

Servings   : _______________

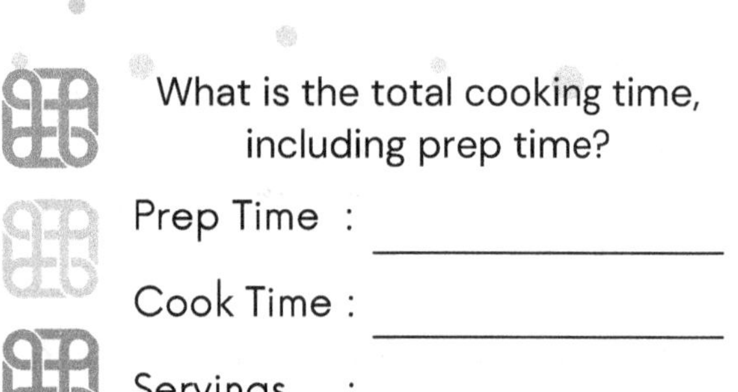

Ingredients:

- 4 boneless, skinless chicken breasts
- 2 tablespoons extra•virgin olive oil
- 3 cloves garlic, minced
- 1 tablespoon chopped fresh rosemary
- 1 teaspoon dried oregano
- Salt and black pepper to taste

Is the recipe easy to follow?

7. Grilled chicken with garlic and herbs

1. Preheat your grill or grill pan to medium•high heat.

2. In a small bowl, combine the olive oil, minced garlic, chopped rosemary, and dried oregano. Season with a pinch of salt and black pepper.

3. Rub the garlic•herb mixture all over the chicken breasts, making sure to coat them evenly on both sides.

4. Grill the chicken for 5•7 minutes per side, or until it's cooked through and the internal temperature reaches 165°F (75°C).

5. Remove the grilled chicken from the heat and let it rest for 5 minutes before serving.

This grilled chicken dish is an excellent anti•inflammatory option:

- Olive oil is high in anti•inflammatory monounsaturated fats.
- Garlic is a potent anti•inflammatory ingredient.
- Rosemary and oregano are both herbs with strong anti•inflammatory properties.
- Chicken is a lean protein that can help reduce inflammation when consumed in moderation.

Serve the grilled chicken with a side of roasted vegetables or a fresh salad for a complete anti•inflammatory meal. Enjoy the delicious flavors of the garlic and herbs while supporting your body's natural inflammatory response.

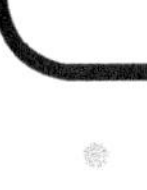

What is the total cooking time, including prep time?

Prep Time : _______________

Cook Time : _______________

Servings : _______________

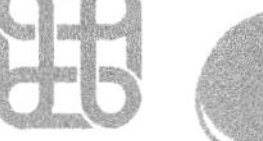 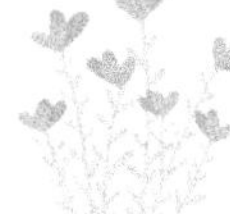

Ingredients:

• 1 bunch of kale, stems removed and leaves chopped
• 2 tablespoons extra•virgin olive oil
• 3 cloves garlic, minced
• 1/4 teaspoon red pepper flakes (optional)
• 1/4 teaspoon sea salt

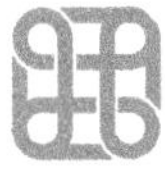 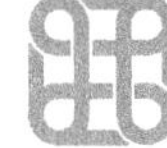 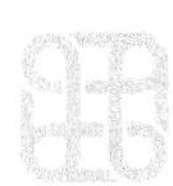 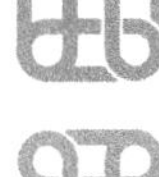 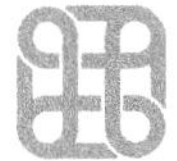

Is the recipe easy to follow?

8. Sautéed kale with garlic

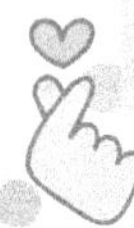

Procedure:

1. In a large skillet or wok, heat the olive oil over medium heat.

2. Add the minced garlic and sauté for 1•2 minutes, or until fragrant.

3. Add the chopped kale leaves to the skillet and toss to coat with the garlic•infused oil.

4. Sprinkle the kale with the red pepper flakes (if using) and sea salt.

5. Sauté the kale for 5•7 minutes, stirring occasionally, until it's wilted and tender.

6. Serve the sautéed kale warm, as a side dish or a topping for grains, proteins, or other vegetables.

This sautéed kale dish is an excellent anti•inflammatory option:

• Kale is a nutrient•dense leafy green that is rich in antioxidants and anti•inflammatory compounds.
• Olive oil is high in anti•inflammatory monounsaturated fats.
• Garlic is a potent anti•inflammatory ingredient.
• Red pepper flakes (if used) can help reduce inflammation due to their capsaicin content.
• Sea salt is a natural anti•inflammatory seasoning.

This simple sautéed kale dish is a great way to incorporate more anti•inflammatory foods into your diet. Enjoy it as a side or incorporate it into other meals for a nutritious and flavorful boost.

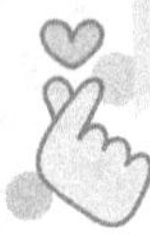

What are the critical points in the recipe (e.g., temperature control, timing)?

What is the total cooking time, including prep time?

Prep Time : _______________

Cook Time : _______________

Servings : _______________

Ingredients:

• 1 cup unsweetened almond milk
• 1 tablespoon matcha green tea powder
• 1 frozen banana
• 1/2 cup frozen spinach
• 1 tablespoon chia seeds

Is the recipe easy to follow?

9. Green tea smoothie bowl

1. In a high•speed blender, combine the almond milk, matcha green tea powder, frozen banana, and frozen spinach.

2. Blend the ingredients on high speed until the mixture is smooth and creamy, about 1•2 minutes.

3. Pour the green tea smoothie into a bowl.

4. Sprinkle the chia seeds over the top of the smoothie.

5. Serve the green tea smoothie bowl immediately, garnished with any additional toppings you desire, such as fresh berries, sliced almonds, or a drizzle of honey.

This green tea smoothie bowl is an excellent anti•inflammatory option:

• Matcha green tea powder is rich in antioxidants and has been shown to have potent anti•inflammatory properties.
• Spinach is a nutrient•dense leafy green that is high in anti•inflammatory compounds.
• Banana provides natural sweetness and fiber, which can help reduce inflammation.
• Almond milk is a dairy•free, low•calorie option that is also anti•inflammatory.
• Chia seeds are a great source of anti•inflammatory omega•3 fatty acids.

This smoothie bowl makes for a refreshing and nourishing breakfast or snack that supports an anti•inflammatory diet. The combination of green tea, leafy greens, and healthy fats provides a powerful anti•inflammatory boost.

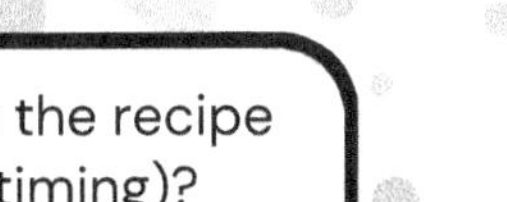
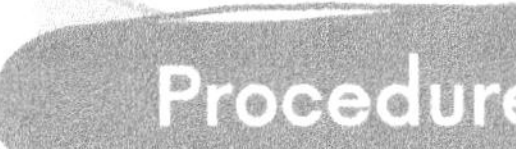

What are the critical points in the recipe (e.g., temperature control, timing)?

What is the total cooking time, including prep time?

Prep Time : _______________

Cook Time : _______________

Servings   : _______________

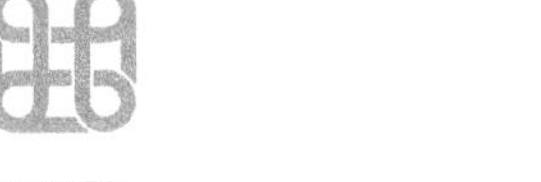
Ingredients:

• 4 cod fillets (about 1 lb total)
• 1 cup cherry tomatoes, halved
• 1/2 cup pitted kalamata olives, halved
• 2 tablespoons extra•virgin olive oil
• 2 cloves garlic, minced
• 1 teaspoon dried oregano
• 1/4 teaspoon red pepper flakes (optional)
• Salt and black pepper to taste

Is the recipe easy to follow?

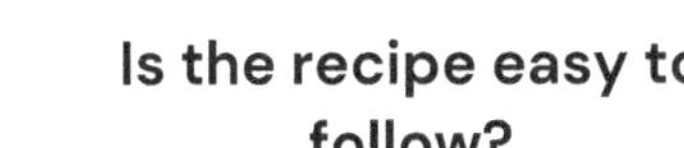
10. Baked cod with tomatoes and olives

1. Preheat your oven to 400°F (200°C).

2. In a baking dish or oven•safe skillet, arrange the cod fillets in a single layer.

3. In a small bowl, combine the cherry tomatoes, olives, olive oil, garlic, oregano, and red pepper flakes (if using). Season with a pinch of salt and black pepper.

4. Spoon the tomato•olive mixture over and around the cod fillets, making sure to distribute it evenly.

5. Bake the cod in the preheated oven for 15•20 minutes, or until the fish is opaque and flakes easily with a fork.

6. Serve the baked cod immediately, spooning the tomato•olive mixture over the top.

This baked cod dish is a delicious and healthy option:

• Cod is a lean, mild•flavored fish that is high in protein and low in mercury.
• Tomatoes are a great source of the antioxidant lycopene, which has anti•inflammatory properties.
• Olives and olive oil are rich in anti•inflammatory monounsaturated fats.
• Garlic and oregano are both herbs with potent anti•inflammatory benefits.
• The red pepper flakes (if used) can help reduce inflammation due to their capsaicin content.

Serve this baked cod with a side of roasted vegetables or a fresh salad for a complete and nutritious meal. Enjoy the bright, Mediterranean•inspired flavors of this simple and delicious dish.

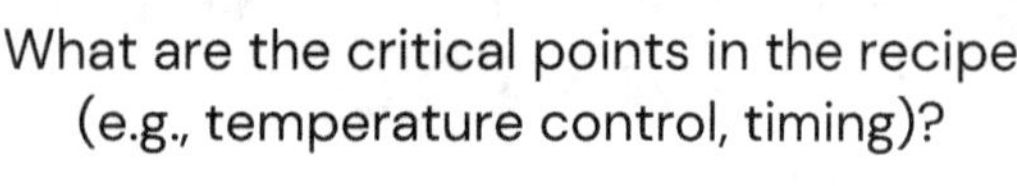

What are the critical points in the recipe (e.g., temperature control, timing)?

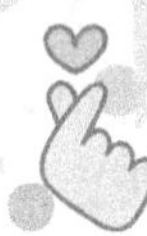

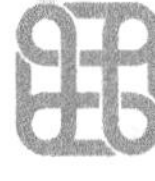

What is the total cooking time, including prep time?

Prep Time : _______________

Cook Time : _______________

Servings   : _______________

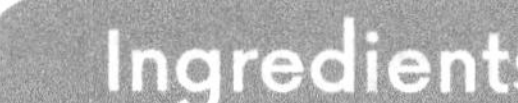

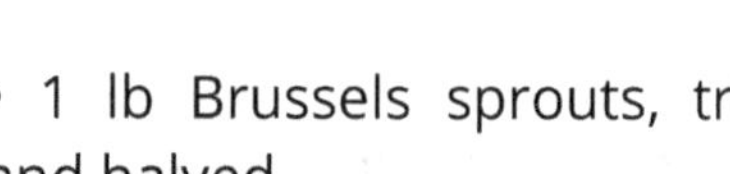

Ingredients:

• 1 lb Brussels sprouts, trimmed and halved
• 2 tablespoons extra•virgin olive oil
• 1 teaspoon garlic powder
• 1/2 teaspoon sea salt
• 1/4 teaspoon ground black pepper

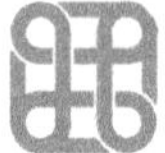
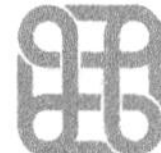
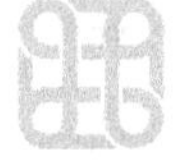
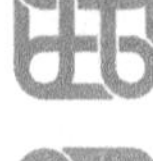
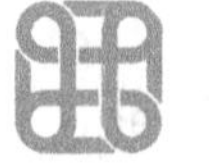

Is the recipe easy to follow?

11. Roasted Brussels sprouts with olive oil

1. Preheat your oven to 400°F (200°C).

2. In a large bowl, toss the trimmed and halved Brussels sprouts with the extra•virgin olive oil, garlic powder, sea salt, and ground black pepper until the sprouts are evenly coated.

3. Spread the seasoned Brussels sprouts in a single layer on a baking sheet.

4. Roast the Brussels sprouts in the preheated oven for 20•25 minutes, or until they are tender and lightly browned on the edges, stirring halfway through.

5. Remove the roasted Brussels sprouts from the oven and serve immediately.

This simple roasted Brussels sprouts dish is an excellent anti•inflammatory option:

• Brussels sprouts are a cruciferous vegetable that is rich in antioxidants and anti•inflammatory compounds.
• Olive oil is high in anti•inflammatory monounsaturated fats.
• Garlic powder is a potent anti•inflammatory ingredient.
• Sea salt and black pepper are natural anti•inflammatory seasonings.

Roasting the Brussels sprouts in olive oil helps to bring out their natural sweetness and enhances the anti•inflammatory benefits of this dish. Serve the roasted Brussels sprouts as a side dish or incorporate them into other meals for a nutritious and flavorful boost.

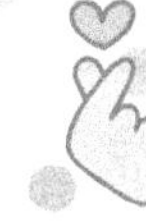

Procedure:

1. In a bowl, place the plain Greek yogurt.

2. Sprinkle the chopped walnuts over the top of the yogurt.

3. Drizzle the honey over the walnuts and yogurt.

4. Gently stir the ingredients together until well combined.

That's it! This simple 3•ingredient dish makes for a delicious and nutritious snack or breakfast.

Here's why this Greek yogurt with walnuts and honey is a great option:

• Greek yogurt is high in protein and probiotics, which can help reduce inflammation.
• Walnuts are a great source of anti•inflammatory omega•3 fatty acids.
• Honey is a natural sweetener that has been shown to have anti•inflammatory properties.

The combination of the creamy Greek yogurt, crunchy walnuts, and sweet honey creates a satisfying and healthy treat. You can adjust the amounts of each ingredient to suit your taste preferences.

This Greek yogurt dish is a versatile option that can be enjoyed for breakfast, as a snack, or even as a light dessert. It's a simple and delicious way to incorporate more anti•inflammatory foods into your diet.

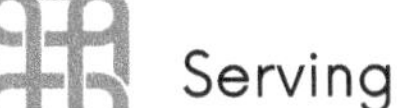

What is the total cooking time, including prep time?

Prep Time : ________________

Cook Time : ________________

Servings   : ________________

Ingredients:

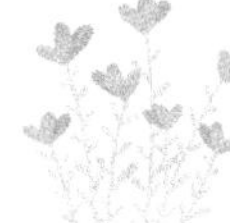

• 1 cup plain Greek yogurt
• 2 tablespoons chopped walnuts
• 1 tablespoon honey

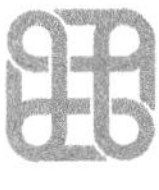
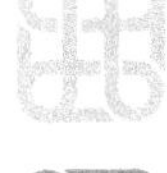
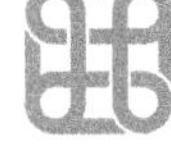
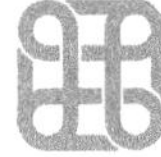
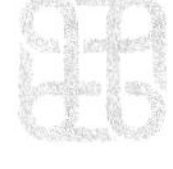
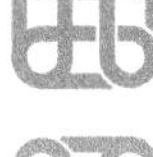
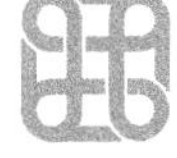

Is the recipe easy to follow?

12. Greek yogurt with walnuts and honey

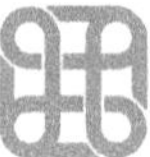

What is the total cooking time, including prep time?

Prep Time : _______________

Cook Time : _______________

Servings   : _______________

Ingredients:

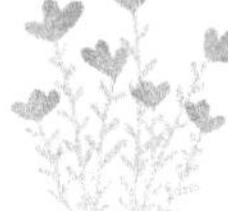

• 1 cup cooked quinoa, cooled
• 1 cup diced cucumber
• 2 tablespoons freshly squeezed lemon juice
• 1 tablespoon extra•virgin olive oil
• 1/4 teaspoon ground black pepper

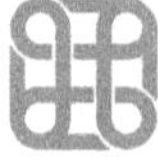
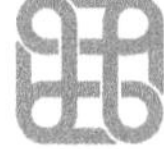
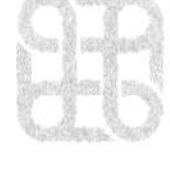
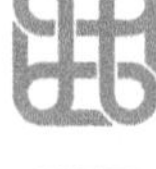
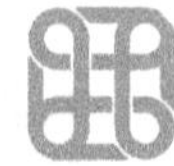

Is the recipe easy to follow?

13. Quinoa salad with cucumber and lemon

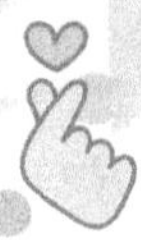

Procedure:

1. In a medium bowl, combine the cooked and cooled quinoa, diced cucumber, lemon juice, olive oil, and black pepper.

2. Toss all the ingredients together until well mixed.

3. Taste and adjust seasoning as needed, adding more lemon juice, olive oil, or black pepper to your preference.

4. Serve the quinoa salad chilled or at room temperature.

This quinoa salad is an excellent anti•inflammatory option for several reasons:

• Quinoa is a nutrient•dense grain that is high in anti•inflammatory antioxidants.
• Cucumbers are a hydrating vegetable that contains anti•inflammatory compounds.
• Lemon juice is a rich source of vitamin C, which has been shown to have anti•inflammatory properties.
• Olive oil is high in anti•inflammatory monounsaturated fats.
• Black pepper contains piperine, a compound with potent anti•inflammatory effects.

This simple quinoa salad makes for a refreshing and nourishing side dish or light meal. The bright flavors of lemon and cucumber pair perfectly with the nutty quinoa. Enjoy this salad as part of an anti•inflammatory diet or as a healthy addition to your meal rotation.

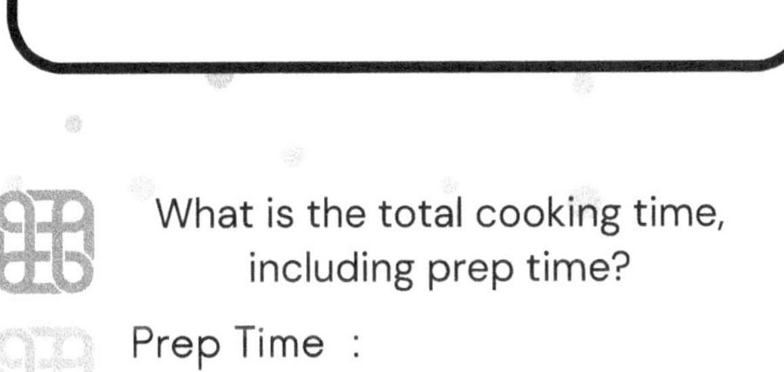

What are the critical points in the recipe (e.g., temperature control, timing)?

What is the total cooking time, including prep time?

Prep Time : _______________

Cook Time : _______________

Servings   : _______________

- 4 large portobello mushroom caps, stems removed
- 2 tablespoons extra•virgin olive oil
- 1 tablespoon balsamic vinegar
- 2 cloves garlic, minced
- 1/2 teaspoon dried thyme

Is the recipe easy to follow?

14. Grilled portobello mushrooms

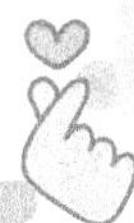

1. Preheat your grill or grill pan to medium•high heat.

2. In a shallow dish, whisk together the olive oil, balsamic vinegar, minced garlic, and dried thyme.

3. Add the portobello mushroom caps to the dish and turn to coat them evenly in the marinade.

4. Grill the marinated portobello mushrooms for 4•5 minutes per side, or until they are tender and slightly charred.

5. Remove the grilled portobello mushrooms from the heat and serve immediately.

This grilled portobello mushroom dish is an excellent anti•inflammatory option:

- Portobello mushrooms are a rich source of antioxidants and anti•inflammatory compounds.
- Olive oil is high in anti•inflammatory monounsaturated fats.
- Balsamic vinegar contains polyphenols that can help reduce inflammation.
- Garlic is a potent anti•inflammatory ingredient.
- Thyme is an herb with strong anti•inflammatory properties.

The simple marinade and grilling method help to bring out the natural umami flavors of the portobello mushrooms while also providing an anti•inflammatory boost. Serve these grilled portobellos as a main dish, or use them as a flavorful topping for salads, grain bowls, or other meals.

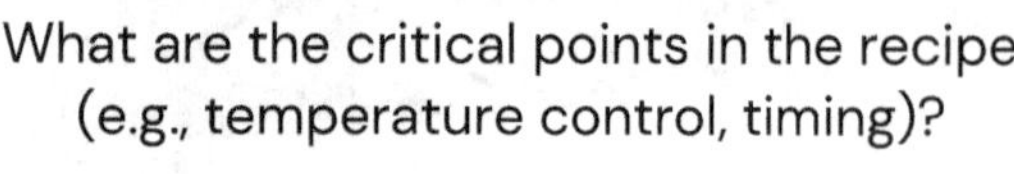

What are the critical points in the recipe (e.g., temperature control, timing)?

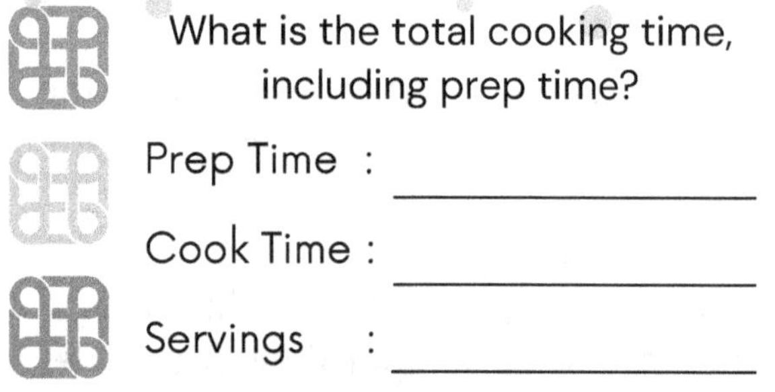

What is the total cooking time, including prep time?

Prep Time : _______________

Cook Time : _______________

Servings : _______________

Ingredients:

- 1 cup old•fashioned rolled oats
- 1 cup unsweetened almond milk
- 1/2 cup fresh or frozen blueberries
- 1 tablespoon chia seeds
- 1 tablespoon sliced almonds

Is the recipe easy to follow?

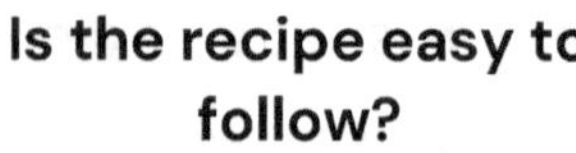

15. Blueberry and almond overnight oats

Procedure:

1. In a medium•sized bowl or mason jar, combine the rolled oats and unsweetened almond milk. Stir to mix well.

2. Gently fold in the fresh or frozen blueberries, chia seeds, and sliced almonds.

3. Cover the bowl or seal the mason jar and refrigerate the overnight oats for at least 4 hours, or overnight.

4. When ready to serve, give the overnight oats a stir to combine the ingredients. You can enjoy them chilled or gently warmed.

This blueberry and almond overnight oats recipe is an excellent anti•inflammatory option:

- Oats are a whole grain that is high in anti•inflammatory fiber.
- Blueberries are a rich source of antioxidants and have potent anti•inflammatory properties.
- Almond milk is a dairy•free, low•calorie option that is also anti•inflammatory.
- Chia seeds are a great source of anti•inflammatory omega•3 fatty acids.
- Almonds are a nutrient•dense nut that contains anti•inflammatory compounds.

The combination of these anti•inflammatory ingredients makes this overnight oats dish a nourishing and delicious breakfast or snack. Enjoy it as a make•ahead option for busy mornings or as a healthy treat any time of day.

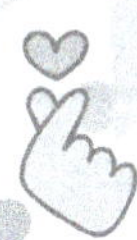

What are the critical points in the recipe (e.g., temperature control, timing)?

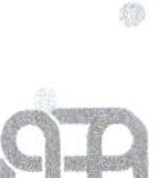

What is the total cooking time, including prep time?

Prep Time : _______________

Cook Time : _______________

Servings : _______________

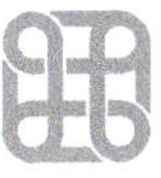 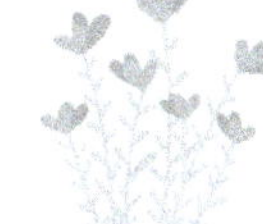

Ingredients:

• 1 block (14 oz) extra•firm tofu, pressed and cut into 1•inch cubes
• 2 tablespoons low•sodium soy sauce
• 1 tablespoon freshly grated ginger
• 1 tablespoon sesame oil
• 1 teaspoon honey (or maple syrup for a vegan option)

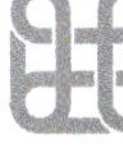
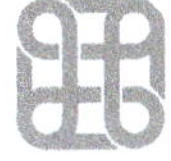
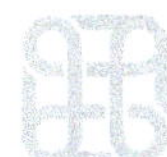
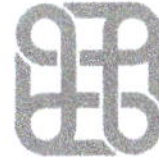
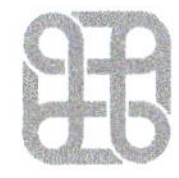

Is the recipe easy to follow?

16. Baked tofu with ginger and soy sauce

1. Preheat your oven to 400°F (200°C). Line a baking sheet with parchment paper.

2. In a medium bowl, whisk together the soy sauce, grated ginger, sesame oil, and honey (or maple syrup).

3. Add the pressed and cubed tofu to the bowl and gently toss to coat the tofu evenly with the marinade.

4. Arrange the marinated tofu cubes in a single layer on the prepared baking sheet.

5. Bake the tofu for 20•25 minutes, flipping the cubes halfway through, until they are golden brown and crispy.

6. Remove the baked tofu from the oven and serve immediately, or allow to cool slightly before serving.

This baked tofu dish is an excellent anti•inflammatory option:

• Tofu is a plant•based protein that is low in inflammatory compounds.
• Ginger is a powerful anti•inflammatory ingredient.
• Soy sauce (use low•sodium) provides flavor without excessive sodium.
• Sesame oil is rich in anti•inflammatory monounsaturated fats.
• Honey (or maple syrup) provides a natural sweetener without the inflammatory effects of refined sugar.

Serve the baked tofu as a main dish, or use it as a protein•packed addition to salads, grain bowls, or stir•fries. This simple recipe is a great way to incorporate more anti•inflammatory foods into your diet.

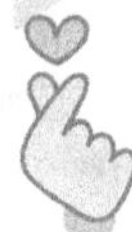

What are the critical points in the recipe (e.g., temperature control, timing)?

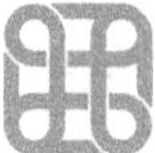 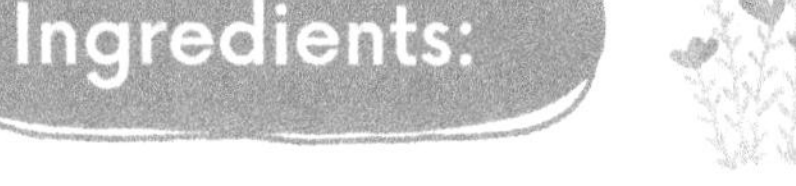

What is the total cooking time, including prep time?

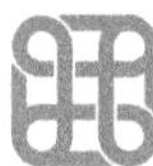
Prep Time : _______________

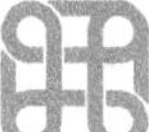
Cook Time : _______________

Servings   : _______________

Ingredients:

• 1 lb carrots, peeled and cut into 1•inch pieces
• 2 tablespoons extra•virgin olive oil
• 1 teaspoon ground cumin
• 1/2 teaspoon ground coriander (optional)
• 1/4 teaspoon sea salt

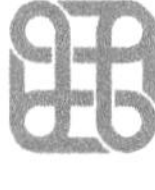 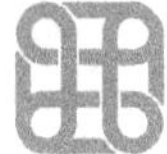 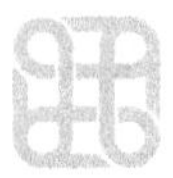 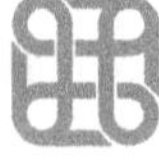 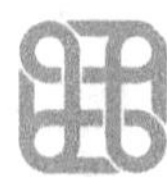

Is the recipe easy to follow?

17. Roasted carrots with cumin

Procedure:

1. Preheat your oven to 400°F (200°C). Line a baking sheet with parchment paper.

2. In a large bowl, toss the peeled and cut carrots with the olive oil, ground cumin, ground coriander (if using), and sea salt until the carrots are evenly coated.

3. Spread the seasoned carrots in a single layer on the prepared baking sheet.

4. Roast the carrots in the preheated oven for 20•25 minutes, or until they are tender and lightly browned, stirring halfway through.

5. Remove the roasted carrots from the oven and serve immediately.

This roasted carrots with cumin dish is an excellent anti•inflammatory option:

• Carrots are a rich source of beta•carotene, an antioxidant with anti•inflammatory properties.
• Olive oil is high in anti•inflammatory monounsaturated fats.
• Cumin is a spice with potent anti•inflammatory effects.
• Coriander (optional) also has anti•inflammatory benefits.
• Sea salt is a natural anti•inflammatory seasoning.

The combination of the sweet, caramelized carrots and the earthy, aromatic spices creates a delicious and nourishing side dish. Enjoy these roasted carrots as a simple accompaniment to grilled proteins or as part of a larger anti•inflammatory meal.

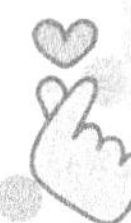

What are the critical points in the recipe (e.g., temperature control, timing)?

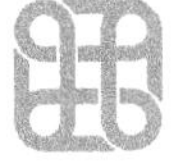
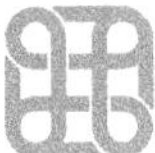

What is the total cooking time, including prep time?

Prep Time : __________________

Cook Time : __________________

Servings   : __________________

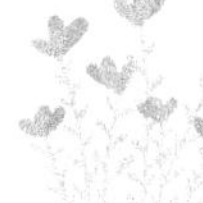

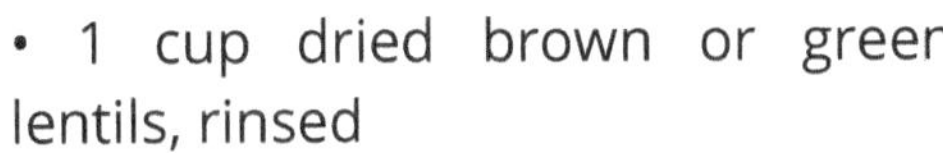

• 1 cup dried brown or green lentils, rinsed
• 4 cups low•sodium vegetable or chicken broth
• 1 tablespoon extra•virgin olive oil
• 1 teaspoon ground turmeric
• 1/2 teaspoon sea salt

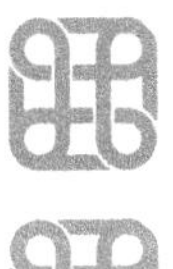
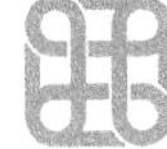

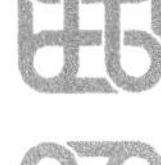
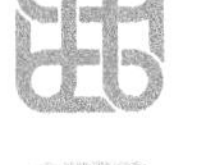

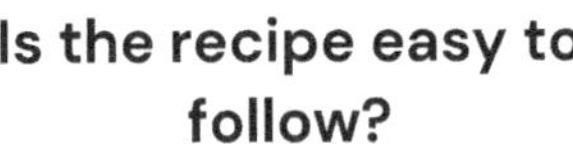
Is the recipe easy to follow?

18. Lentil soup with turmeric

1. In a large pot, combine the rinsed lentils and broth. Bring the mixture to a boil over high heat.

2. Once boiling, reduce the heat to medium•low, cover the pot, and let the lentils simmer for 15•20 minutes, or until they are tender.

3. Stir in the olive oil, ground turmeric, and sea salt. Taste and adjust seasoning as needed.

4. Continue to simmer the lentil soup for an additional 5 minutes to allow the flavors to meld.

5. Serve the lentil soup hot, garnished with additional toppings if desired, such as chopped fresh parsley or a drizzle of olive oil.

This lentil soup with turmeric is an excellent anti•inflammatory option:

• Lentils are a nutrient•dense legume that are high in anti•inflammatory fiber and protein.
• Turmeric is a powerful anti•inflammatory spice due to its active compound, curcumin.
• Olive oil provides anti•inflammatory monounsaturated fats.
• Sea salt is a natural anti•inflammatory seasoning.
• Broth (low•sodium) adds flavor without excessive sodium.

This simple lentil soup is a comforting and nourishing meal that supports an anti•inflammatory diet. Enjoy it as a main dish or as a side to a larger anti•inflammatory meal. The turmeric adds a beautiful golden color and earthy flavor to the soup.

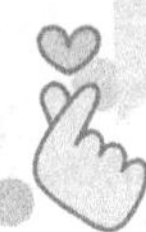

Procedure:

1. In a steamer basket or saucepan with a steamer insert, bring the water to a boil over high heat.

2. Add the broccoli florets to the steamer basket, cover, and steam for 5•7 minutes, or until the broccoli is tender•crisp.

3. Carefully transfer the steamed broccoli to a serving bowl.

4. Drizzle the lemon juice and olive oil over the broccoli, and season with salt and pepper to taste.

5. Toss the broccoli gently to coat it evenly with the lemon and oil.

6. Serve the steamed broccoli with lemon immediately, while it's hot.

This simple steamed broccoli dish is a great option for a few reasons:

• Broccoli is a nutrient•dense cruciferous vegetable that is rich in antioxidants and anti•inflammatory compounds.
• Lemon juice is a good source of vitamin C, which has anti•inflammatory properties.
• Olive oil provides healthy monounsaturated fats that can help reduce inflammation.
• The minimal cooking method of steaming helps to preserve the broccoli's nutrients and natural flavors.

This steamed broccoli with lemon makes for a quick and easy side dish that can be paired with a variety of main courses. The bright, tangy lemon complements the earthy, slightly sweet broccoli perfectly. Enjoy this simple, yet flavorful, vegetable dish as part of a balanced, anti•inflammatory meal.

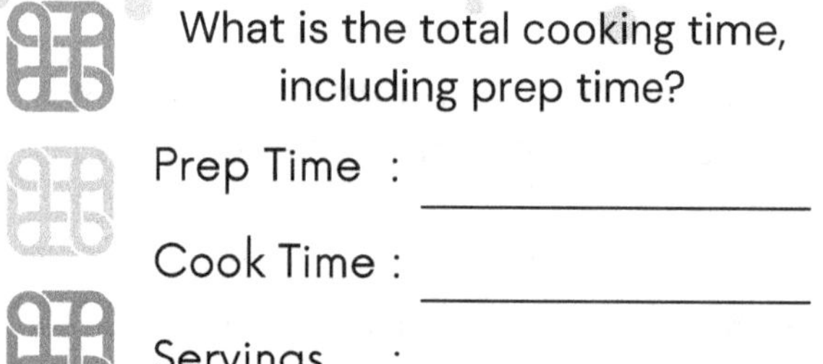

What is the total cooking time, including prep time?

Prep Time   :   _______________

Cook Time :   _______________

Servings   :   _______________

Ingredients:

• 1 lb broccoli florets
• 2 tablespoons water
• 1 tablespoon fresh lemon juice
• 1 teaspoon olive oil
• Salt and pepper to taste

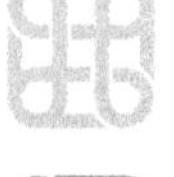
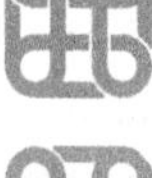

Is the recipe easy to follow?

19. Steamed broccoli with lemon

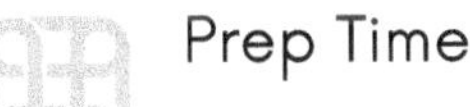
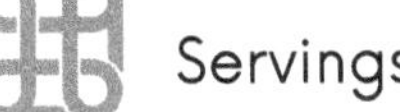

What is the total cooking time, including prep time?

Prep Time : _________________

Cook Time : _________________

Servings : _________________

Ingredients:

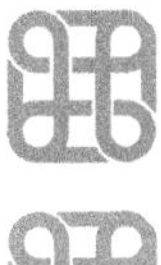
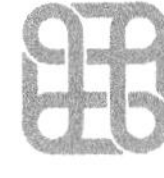
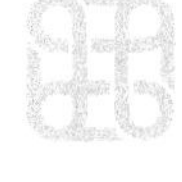

- 4 medium•sized apples, cored and halved
- 2 tablespoons chopped walnuts
- 1 tablespoon honey (or maple syrup for a vegan option)
- 1 teaspoon ground cinnamon
- 1 tablespoon water

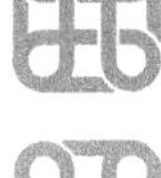
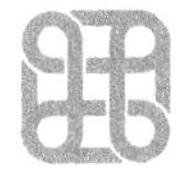

Is the recipe easy to follow?

20. Baked apple with cinnamon and walnuts

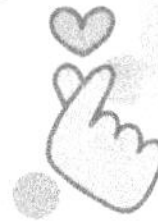

Procedure:

1. Preheat your oven to 375°F (190°C).

2. Place the apple halves in a baking dish or on a parchment•lined baking sheet.

3. In a small bowl, mix together the chopped walnuts, honey (or maple syrup), and ground cinnamon.

4. Spoon the walnut•cinnamon mixture evenly into the center of each apple half.

5. Pour the water into the bottom of the baking dish or around the apples on the baking sheet.

6. Bake the stuffed apples for 20•25 minutes, or until the apples are tender and the filling is lightly browned.

7. Serve the baked apples warm, with any juices spooned over the top.

This baked apple dish is an excellent anti•inflammatory option:

- Apples are a good source of anti•inflammatory antioxidants.
- Walnuts are rich in anti•inflammatory omega•3 fatty acids.
- Cinnamon is a spice with potent anti•inflammatory properties.
- Honey (or maple syrup) provides a natural sweetener without the inflammatory effects of refined sugar.

The combination of the warm, cinnamon•spiced apples and the crunchy, nutty walnuts creates a delightful and nourishing dessert or snack. Enjoy this baked apple dish as a comforting and anti•inflammatory treat.

What are the critical points in the recipe (e.g., temperature control, timing)?

What is the total cooking time, including prep time?

Prep Time : ___________________

Cook Time : ___________________

Servings : ___________________

Ingredients:

• 2 medium zucchini, sliced lengthwise into 1/2•inch thick strips
• 2 tablespoons extra•virgin olive oil
• 1 tablespoon chopped fresh basil
• 1 tablespoon chopped fresh parsley
• 1/4 teaspoon sea salt

Is the recipe easy to follow?

🙂 🙁

21. Grilled zucchini with herbs

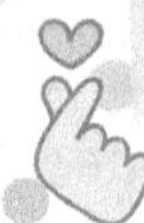

Procedure:

1. Preheat your grill or grill pan to medium•high heat.

2. In a large bowl, toss the zucchini strips with the olive oil, making sure they are evenly coated.

3. Sprinkle the chopped basil, parsley, and sea salt over the oiled zucchini and toss gently to combine.

4. Grill the zucchini strips for 3•4 minutes per side, or until they are tender and have grill marks.

5. Remove the grilled zucchini from the heat and serve immediately, garnished with any additional fresh herbs if desired.

This grilled zucchini dish is an excellent anti•inflammatory option:

• Zucchini is a nutrient•dense vegetable that is rich in antioxidants and anti•inflammatory compounds.
• Olive oil provides healthy monounsaturated fats with anti•inflammatory properties.
• Basil and parsley are herbs with potent anti•inflammatory benefits.
• Sea salt is a natural anti•inflammatory seasoning.

The simple preparation of grilling the zucchini with a few flavorful herbs allows the natural sweetness and texture of the vegetable to shine. Serve this grilled zucchini as a side dish or incorporate it into larger anti•inflammatory meals, such as salads or grain bowls.

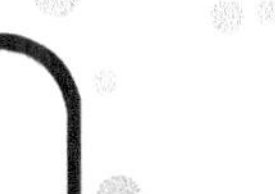

Procedure:

What is the total cooking time, including prep time?

Prep Time : ___________________

Cook Time : ___________________

Servings : ___________________

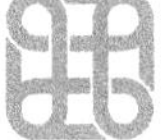
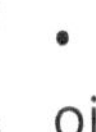
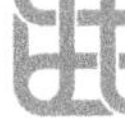
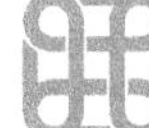
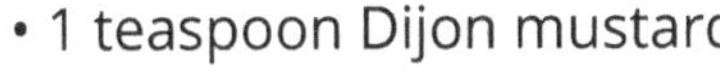
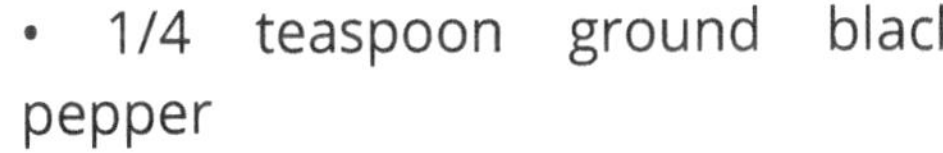

Ingredients:

• 2 (4 oz) cans of sardines in olive oil, drained
• 2 slices of whole grain bread, toasted
• 1 tablespoon lemon juice
• 1 teaspoon Dijon mustard
• 1/4 teaspoon ground black pepper

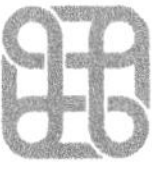
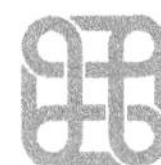
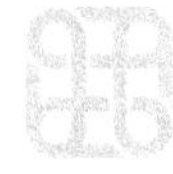
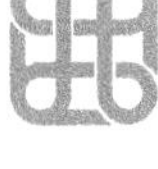
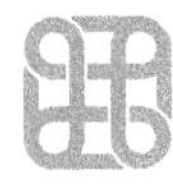

Is the recipe easy to follow?

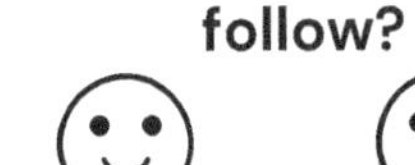

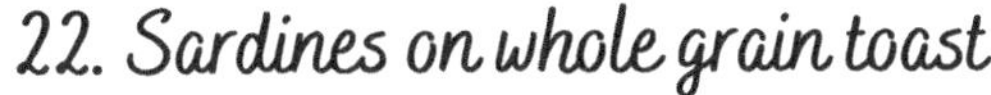

22. Sardines on whole grain toast

1. In a small bowl, gently flake the drained sardines with a fork.

2. Add the lemon juice, Dijon mustard, and ground black pepper to the sardines. Stir to combine.

3. Spread the sardine mixture evenly over the two slices of toasted whole grain bread.

4. Serve the sardine toast immediately.

This sardine toast is an excellent anti•inflammatory option for several reasons:

• Sardines are a fatty fish that are rich in anti•inflammatory omega•3 fatty acids.
• Whole grain bread provides complex carbohydrates and fiber, which can help reduce inflammation.
• Lemon juice is a good source of vitamin C, an antioxidant with anti•inflammatory properties.
• Dijon mustard contains compounds that may have anti•inflammatory effects.
• Black pepper contains piperine, a compound with potent anti•inflammatory benefits.

The combination of the nutrient•dense sardines, whole grain toast, and anti•inflammatory seasonings makes this a simple yet nourishing meal or snack. Sardines are also a sustainable and affordable source of protein and healthy fats.

Enjoy this sardine toast as part of a balanced, anti•inflammatory diet. It's a quick and easy way to incorporate more anti•inflammatory foods into your routine.

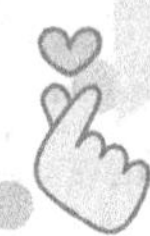

Procedure:

1. Preheat your oven to 400°F (200°C). Line a baking sheet with parchment paper.

2. In a large bowl, toss the bell pepper strips with the olive oil, minced garlic, dried oregano, and sea salt until the peppers are evenly coated.

3. Spread the seasoned bell pepper strips in a single layer on the prepared baking sheet.

4. Roast the bell peppers in the preheated oven for 20•25 minutes, or until they are tender and lightly charred, stirring halfway through.

5. Remove the roasted bell peppers from the oven and serve immediately, while still warm.

This roasted bell pepper dish is an excellent anti•inflammatory option:

• Bell peppers are a rich source of vitamin C, an antioxidant with anti•inflammatory properties.
• Olive oil provides healthy monounsaturated fats that can help reduce inflammation.
• Garlic is a potent anti•inflammatory ingredient.
• Oregano is an herb with strong anti•inflammatory benefits.
• Sea salt is a natural anti•inflammatory seasoning.

The simple roasting method brings out the natural sweetness of the bell peppers, while the garlic and oregano add depth of flavor. Serve these roasted bell peppers as a side dish, or use them as a topping for salads, grain bowls, or other anti•inflammatory meals.

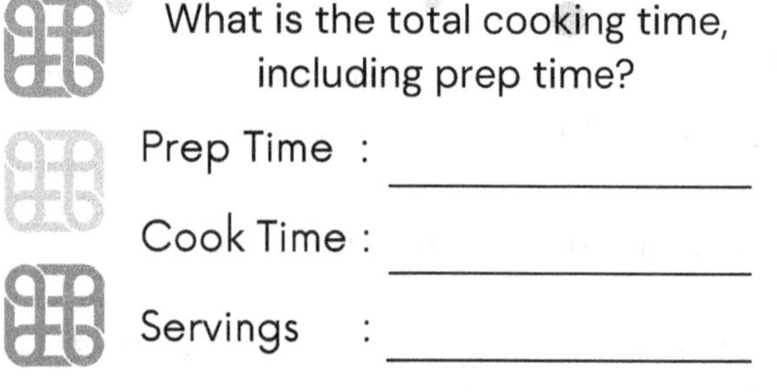

What is the total cooking time, including prep time?

Prep Time : ________________

Cook Time : ________________

Servings   : ________________

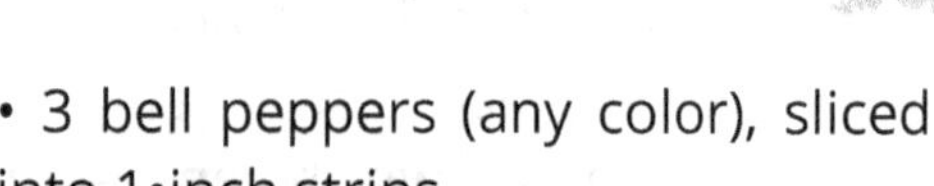

Ingredients:

• 3 bell peppers (any color), sliced into 1•inch strips
• 2 tablespoons extra•virgin olive oil
• 3 cloves garlic, minced
• 1 teaspoon dried oregano
• 1/4 teaspoon sea salt

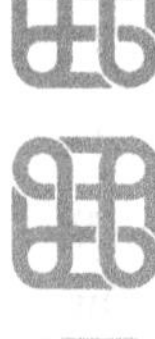
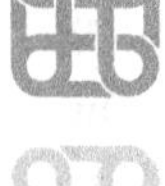
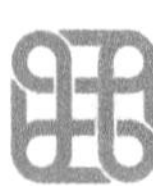
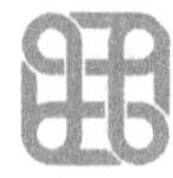

Is the recipe easy to follow?

23. Roasted bell peppers with garlic

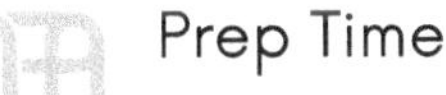
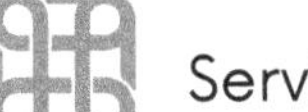

What is the total cooking time, including prep time?

Prep Time : _______________

Cook Time : _______________

Servings : _______________

Ingredients:

- 2 cups fresh spinach leaves
- 2 eggs
- 1 tablespoon white vinegar
- 1 tablespoon extra•virgin olive oil
- 1/4 teaspoon sea salt

Is the recipe easy to follow?

24. Poached eggs on spinach

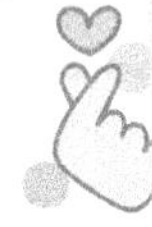

Procedure:

1. In a medium saucepan, bring 3•4 inches of water to a gentle simmer over medium heat. Add the white vinegar.

2. Crack the eggs one at a time into a small bowl or cup, then gently slide them into the simmering water. Poach the eggs for 3•5 minutes, or until the whites are set but the yolks are still runny.

3. While the eggs are poaching, heat the olive oil in a small skillet over medium heat. Add the fresh spinach leaves and sauté for 1•2 minutes, just until the spinach is wilted.

4. Remove the poached eggs from the water using a slotted spoon and place them on top of the sautéed spinach.

5. Sprinkle the poached eggs and spinach with the sea salt.

6. Serve the poached eggs on spinach immediately.

This poached egg and spinach dish is an excellent anti•inflammatory option:

- Spinach is a nutrient•dense leafy green that is rich in antioxidants and anti•inflammatory compounds.
- Eggs are a high•quality protein source that can help reduce inflammation.
- Olive oil provides healthy monounsaturated fats with anti•inflammatory properties.
- Vinegar contains acetic acid, which may have anti•inflammatory effects.
- Sea salt is a natural anti•inflammatory seasoning.

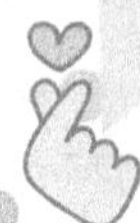

Procedure:

What is the total cooking time, including prep time?

Prep Time : _______________

Cook Time : _______________

Servings : _______________

Ingredients:

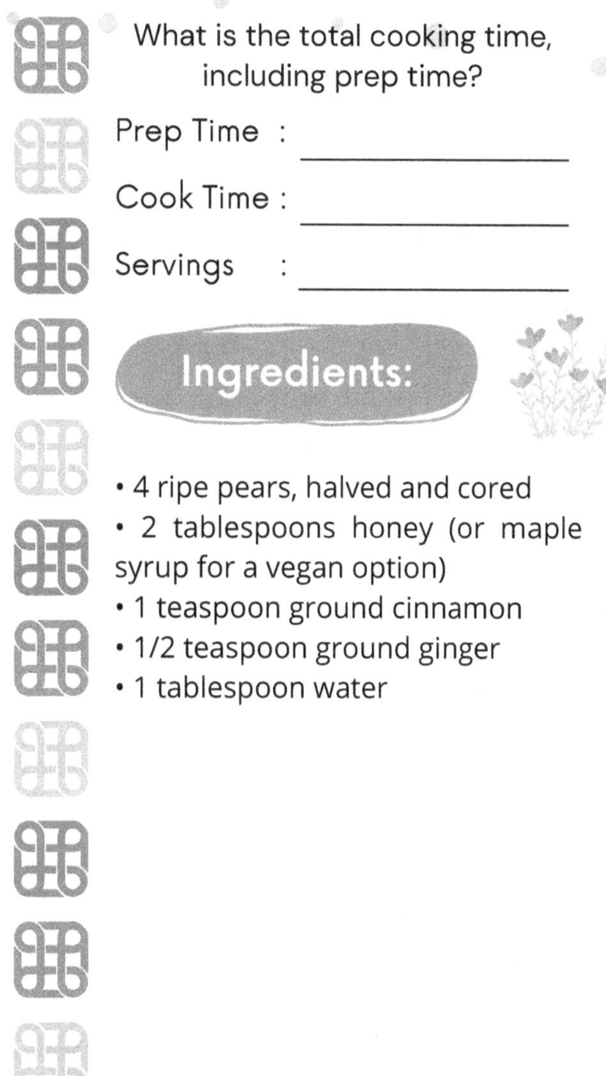

- 4 ripe pears, halved and cored
- 2 tablespoons honey (or maple syrup for a vegan option)
- 1 teaspoon ground cinnamon
- 1/2 teaspoon ground ginger
- 1 tablespoon water

Is the recipe easy to follow?

☺   ☹

25. Baked pear with cinnamon and ginger

1. Preheat your oven to 375°F (190°C).

2. Place the pear halves, cut•side up, in a baking dish or on a parchment•lined baking sheet.

3. In a small bowl, mix together the honey (or maple syrup), ground cinnamon, and ground ginger.

4. Spoon the cinnamon•ginger mixture evenly over the pear halves, making sure to coat the tops and sides.

5. Pour the water into the bottom of the baking dish or around the pears on the baking sheet.

6. Bake the pears for 20•25 minutes, or until they are tender when pierced with a fork.

7. Remove the baked pears from the oven and serve warm, with any juices spooned over the top.

This baked pear dish is a great option for an anti•inflammatory diet:

- Pears are a fruit that are high in antioxidants and anti•inflammatory compounds.
- Cinnamon is a spice with potent anti•inflammatory properties.
- Ginger is another spice with strong anti•inflammatory benefits.
- Honey (or maple syrup) provides a natural sweetener without the inflammatory effects of refined sugar.

The combination of the warm, spiced pears and the natural sweetness creates a comforting and nourishing dessert or snack. Enjoy these baked pears on their own or serve them with a dollop of plain Greek yogurt for an extra boost of protein.

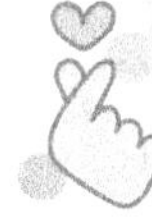

Procedure:

What is the total cooking time, including prep time?

Prep Time : _________________

Cook Time : _________________

Servings   : _________________

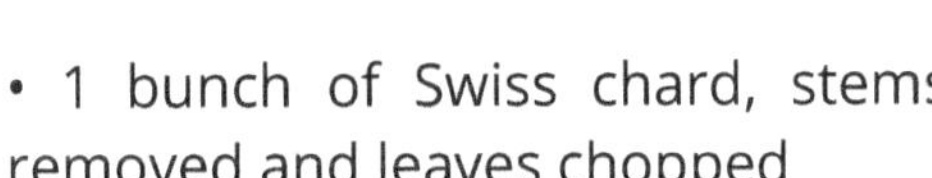

Ingredients:

• 1 bunch of Swiss chard, stems removed and leaves chopped
• 2 tablespoons extra•virgin olive oil
• 3 cloves garlic, minced
• 1/4 teaspoon red pepper flakes (optional)
• 1/4 teaspoon sea salt

Is the recipe easy to follow?

26. Sautéed Swiss chard with garlic

1. In a large skillet or wok, heat the olive oil over medium heat.

2. Add the minced garlic to the skillet and sauté for 1•2 minutes, or until fragrant.

3. Add the chopped Swiss chard leaves to the skillet and toss to coat with the garlic•infused oil.

4. Sprinkle the chard with the red pepper flakes (if using) and sea salt.

5. Sauté the Swiss chard for 5•7 minutes, stirring occasionally, until the leaves are wilted and tender.

6. Serve the sautéed Swiss chard warm, as a side dish or a topping for grains, proteins, or other vegetables.

This sautéed Swiss chard dish is a great option for an anti•inflammatory diet:

• Swiss chard is a nutrient•dense leafy green that is rich in antioxidants and anti•inflammatory compounds.
• Olive oil provides healthy monounsaturated fats with anti•inflammatory properties.
• Garlic is a potent anti•inflammatory ingredient.
• Red pepper flakes (if used) can help reduce inflammation due to their capsaicin content.
• Sea salt is a natural anti•inflammatory seasoning.

The simple sautéing method helps to preserve the chard's nutrients and natural flavors. Serve this dish as a side or incorporate it into other anti•inflammatory meals for a nutritious and flavorful boost.

What are the critical points in the recipe (e.g., temperature control, timing)?

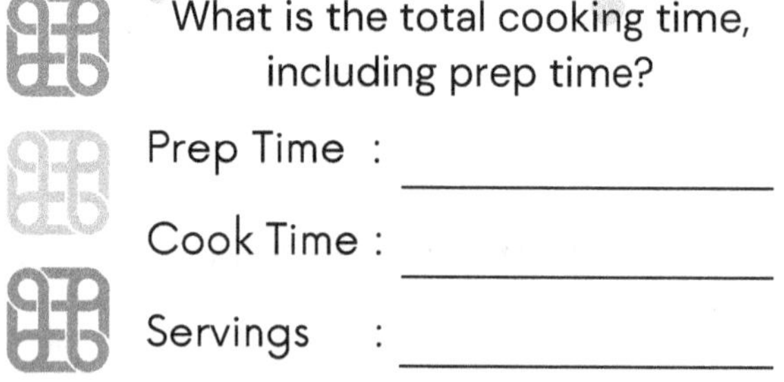

What is the total cooking time, including prep time?

Prep Time : ________________

Cook Time : ________________

Servings   : ________________

• 1 lb large shrimp, peeled and deveined
• 2 tablespoons extra•virgin olive oil
• 2 tablespoons freshly squeezed lemon juice
• 2 cloves garlic, minced
• 1 tablespoon chopped fresh parsley
• 1 teaspoon dried oregano
• 1/4 teaspoon sea salt
• 1/4 teaspoon ground black pepper

Is the recipe easy to follow?

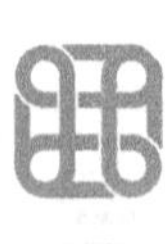
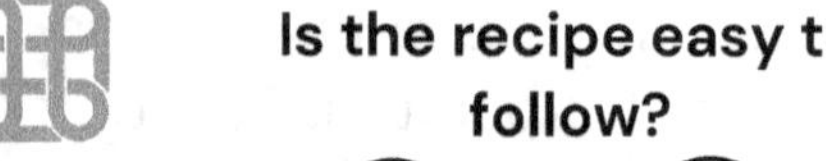

27. Grilled shrimp with lemon and herbs

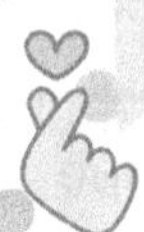

1. In a large bowl, combine the shrimp, olive oil, lemon juice, minced garlic, chopped parsley, dried oregano, sea salt, and black pepper. Toss to coat the shrimp evenly.

2. Preheat your grill or grill pan to medium•high heat.

3. Thread the marinated shrimp onto skewers, if desired, for easier handling on the grill.

4. Grill the shrimp for 2•3 minutes per side, or until they are opaque and cooked through.

5. Remove the grilled shrimp from the heat and serve immediately, garnished with additional lemon wedges and chopped parsley if desired.

This grilled shrimp dish is a great option for an anti•inflammatory diet:

• Shrimp is a lean protein that is low in inflammatory compounds.
• Olive oil provides healthy monounsaturated fats with anti•inflammatory properties.
• Lemon juice is a good source of vitamin C, an antioxidant with anti•inflammatory benefits.
• Garlic and herbs like parsley and oregano have potent anti•inflammatory effects.
• Sea salt and black pepper are natural anti•inflammatory seasonings.

The bright, zesty flavors of the lemon, herbs, and garlic complement the grilled shrimp perfectly. Serve this dish as a main course or use the shrimp as a protein•packed addition to salads, grain bowls, or other anti•inflammatory meals.

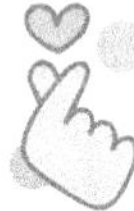

Procedure:

1. Preheat your oven to 400°F (200°C). Line a baking sheet with parchment paper.

2. In a large bowl, toss the sweet potato wedges with the olive oil, cumin, smoked paprika, sea salt, and black pepper until the potatoes are evenly coated.

3. Spread the seasoned sweet potato wedges in a single layer on the prepared baking sheet.

4. Roast the sweet potatoes in the preheated oven for 25•30 minutes, flipping them halfway through, until they are tender and lightly browned.

5. Remove the roasted sweet potato wedges from the oven and serve immediately, while hot.

This roasted sweet potato dish is a great option for an anti•inflammatory diet:

• Sweet potatoes are a nutrient•dense root vegetable that are high in anti•inflammatory antioxidants, such as beta•carotene.
• Olive oil provides healthy monounsaturated fats with anti•inflammatory properties.
• Cumin and smoked paprika are spices with potent anti•inflammatory benefits.
• Sea salt and black pepper are natural anti•inflammatory seasonings.

The combination of the sweet, caramelized potatoes and the earthy, aromatic spices creates a delicious and nourishing side dish. Enjoy these roasted sweet potato wedges as a simple accompaniment to grilled proteins or as part of a larger anti•inflammatory meal.

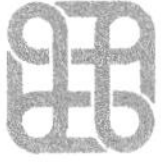

What is the total cooking time, including prep time?

Prep Time : _________________

Cook Time : _________________

Servings   : _________________

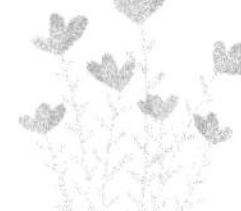

Ingredients:

• 2 lbs sweet potatoes, peeled and cut into 1•inch wedges
• 2 tablespoons extra•virgin olive oil
• 1 teaspoon ground cumin
• 1/2 teaspoon smoked paprika
• 1/2 teaspoon sea salt
• 1/4 teaspoon ground black pepper

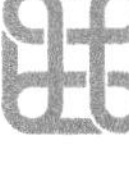
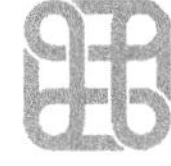
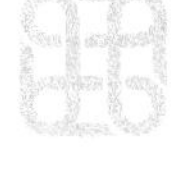
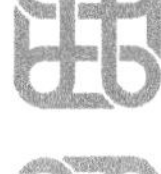
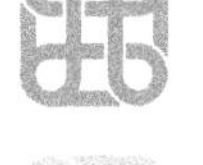

Is the recipe easy to follow?

28. Roasted sweet potato wedges

What is the total cooking time, including prep time?

Prep Time : _______________

Cook Time : _______________

Servings : _______________

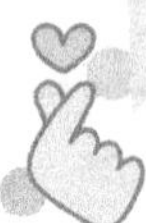

Ingredients:

• 1 cup fresh spinach leaves
• 1 ripe banana, frozen
• 1 cup unsweetened almond milk
• 1 tablespoon ground flaxseed
• 1 teaspoon honey (or maple syrup for a vegan option)

Is the recipe easy to follow?

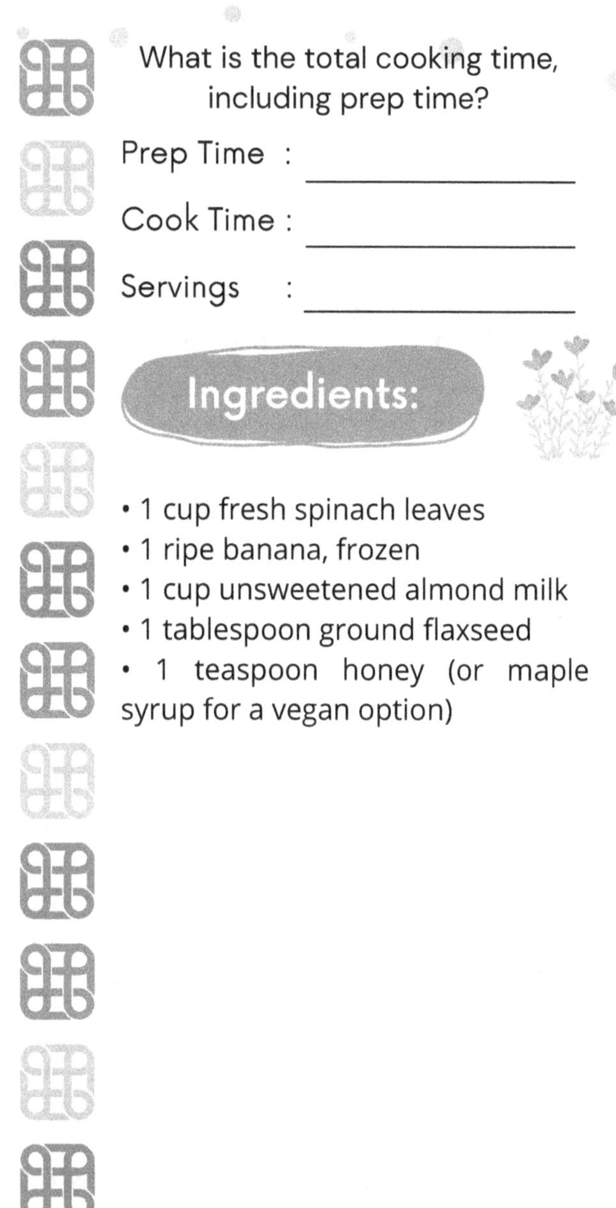

29. Green smoothie with spinach and banana

Procedure:

1. In a high•speed blender, combine the fresh spinach leaves, frozen banana, almond milk, ground flaxseed, and honey (or maple syrup).

2. Blend the ingredients on high speed until the mixture is smooth and creamy, about 1•2 minutes.

3. Pour the green smoothie into a glass and enjoy immediately.

This green smoothie is an excellent anti•inflammatory option:

• Spinach is a nutrient•dense leafy green that is rich in antioxidants and anti•inflammatory compounds.
• Bananas provide natural sweetness and fiber, which can help reduce inflammation.
• Almond milk is a dairy•free, low•calorie option that is also anti•inflammatory.
• Flaxseed is a great source of anti•inflammatory omega•3 fatty acids.
• Honey (or maple syrup) provides a natural sweetener without the inflammatory effects of refined sugar.

The combination of the leafy greens, fruit, and healthy fats creates a nourishing and delicious smoothie that supports an anti•inflammatory diet. This green smoothie makes for a quick and easy breakfast or snack that can be enjoyed year•round.

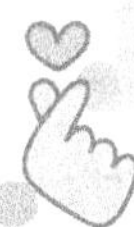

Procedure:

1. Preheat your oven to 400°F (200°C). Line a baking sheet with parchment paper.

2. Place the salmon fillets on the prepared baking sheet.

3. In a small bowl, whisk together the olive oil, lemon juice, and chopped dill.

4. Drizzle the dill•lemon mixture evenly over the salmon fillets, making sure to coat them well.

5. Sprinkle the salmon with the sea salt.

6. Bake the salmon in the preheated oven for 12•15 minutes, or until it flakes easily with a fork and is cooked through.

7. Serve the baked salmon warm, garnished with additional fresh dill if desired.

This baked salmon dish is an excellent anti•inflammatory option:

• Salmon is a fatty fish that is rich in anti•inflammatory omega•3 fatty acids.
• Olive oil provides healthy monounsaturated fats with anti•inflammatory properties.
• Lemon juice is a good source of vitamin C, an antioxidant with anti•inflammatory benefits.
• Dill is an herb with potent anti•inflammatory compounds.
• Sea salt is a natural anti•inflammatory seasoning.

The simple preparation of baking the salmon with the bright, herbal flavors of dill and lemon creates a delicious and nourishing meal. Serve this salmon with roasted vegetables or a fresh salad for a complete anti•inflammatory dinner.

What is the total cooking time, including prep time?

Prep Time : ______________

Cook Time : ______________

Servings : ______________

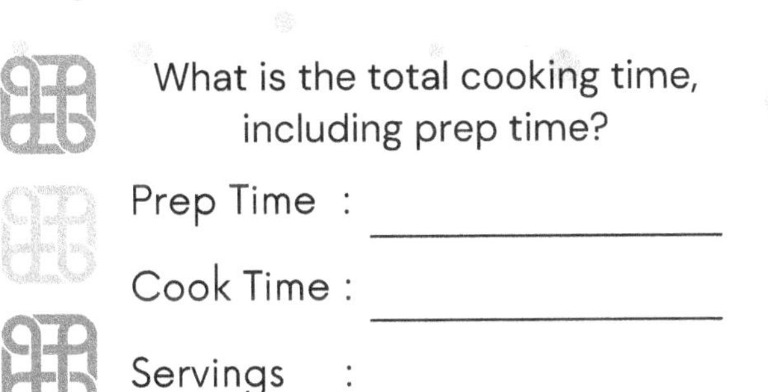

Ingredients:

• 4 (6 oz) salmon fillets
• 2 tablespoons extra•virgin olive oil
• 2 tablespoons freshly squeezed lemon juice
• 2 tablespoons chopped fresh dill
• 1/4 teaspoon sea salt

Is the recipe easy to follow?

30. Baked salmon with dill and lemon

What are the critical points in the recipe (e.g., temperature control, timing)?

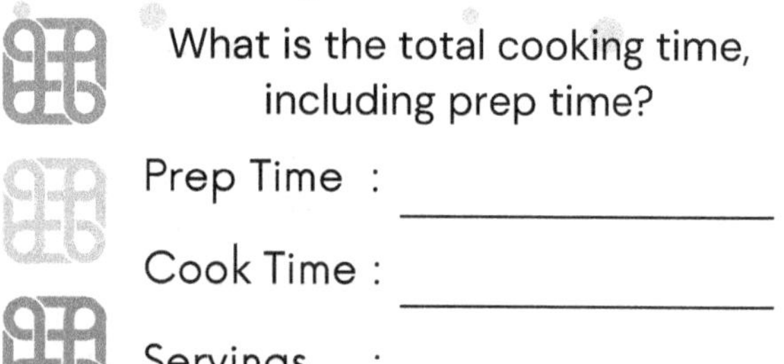

What is the total cooking time, including prep time?

Prep Time : _______________

Cook Time : _______________

Servings   : _______________

Ingredients:

- 1 lb asparagus, trimmed
- 2 tablespoons water
- 1 tablespoon extra•virgin olive oil
- 1 clove garlic, minced
- 1/4 teaspoon sea salt

Is the recipe easy to follow?

31. Steamed asparagus with olive oil

Procedure:

1. In a steamer basket or saucepan with a steamer insert, bring the water to a boil over high heat.

2. Add the trimmed asparagus spears to the steamer basket, cover, and steam for 5•7 minutes, or until the asparagus is tender•crisp.

3. Carefully transfer the steamed asparagus to a serving bowl.

4. Drizzle the olive oil over the asparagus and sprinkle with the minced garlic and sea salt.

5. Toss the asparagus gently to coat it evenly with the olive oil, garlic, and salt. Serve the steamed asparagus with olive oil immediately, while it's hot.

This simple steamed asparagus dish is an excellent anti•inflammatory option:

• Asparagus is a nutrient•dense vegetable that is rich in antioxidants and anti•inflammatory compounds.
• Olive oil provides healthy monounsaturated fats with anti•inflammatory properties.
• Garlic is a potent anti•inflammatory ingredient.
• Sea salt is a natural anti•inflammatory seasoning.

The minimal cooking method of steaming helps to preserve the asparagus's nutrients and natural flavors. The addition of the olive oil, garlic, and sea salt enhances the dish's anti•inflammatory benefits.

Serve this steamed asparagus with olive oil as a side dish or incorporate it into other anti•inflammatory meals. It's a quick and easy way to add more nutrient•dense, anti•inflammatory vegetables to your diet.

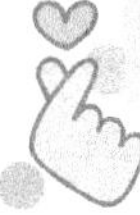

Procedure:

2. Let the mixture sit for 10•15 minutes, stirring occasionally, until the chia seeds have formed a gel•like consistency.

3. Stir in the lemon juice and honey (if using). Add a pinch of turmeric for extra anti•inflammatory benefits.

4. Refrigerate for at least 30 minutes to allow the flavors to meld.

5. Enjoy the chia seed water chilled. You can sip it throughout the day.

The chia seeds provide fiber, omega•3s, and antioxidants. The lemon adds vitamin C, which has anti•inflammatory properties. The optional honey and turmeric also have anti•inflammatory effects.

This simple 5•ingredient drink is a great way to stay hydrated and support your body's natural inflammatory response.

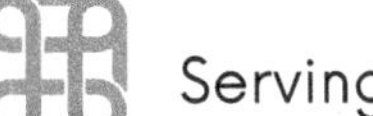

What is the total cooking time, including prep time?

Prep Time : _________________

Cook Time : _________________

Servings : _________________

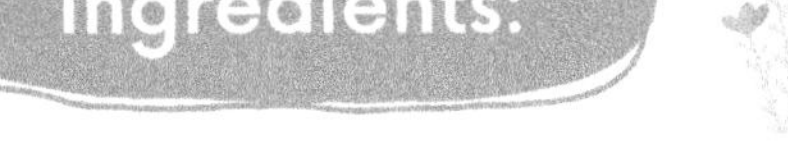

Ingredients:

• 2 tbsp chia seeds
• 4 cups water
• 1 lemon, juiced
• 1 tsp honey (optional)
• Pinch of ground turmeric (optional)

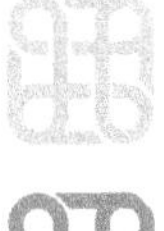
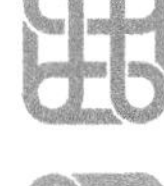
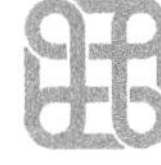
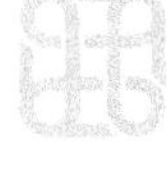
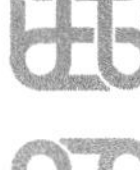
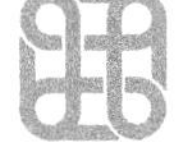

Is the recipe easy to follow?

32. Chia seed water with lemon

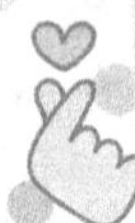

1. Preheat grill or grill pan to medium•high heat.

2. Brush the eggplant slices on both sides with olive oil. Season with salt, pepper, oregano, and basil.

3. Grill the eggplant slices for 3•4 minutes per side, or until tender and charred in spots.

4. Serve the grilled eggplant immediately, garnished with extra herbs if desired.

That's it! The key is to use high•quality, fresh eggplant and simple seasonings to let the natural flavors shine. Enjoy this easy and delicious grilled eggplant dish.

What is the total cooking time, including prep time?

Prep Time : _______________

Cook Time : _______________

Servings : _______________

Ingredients:

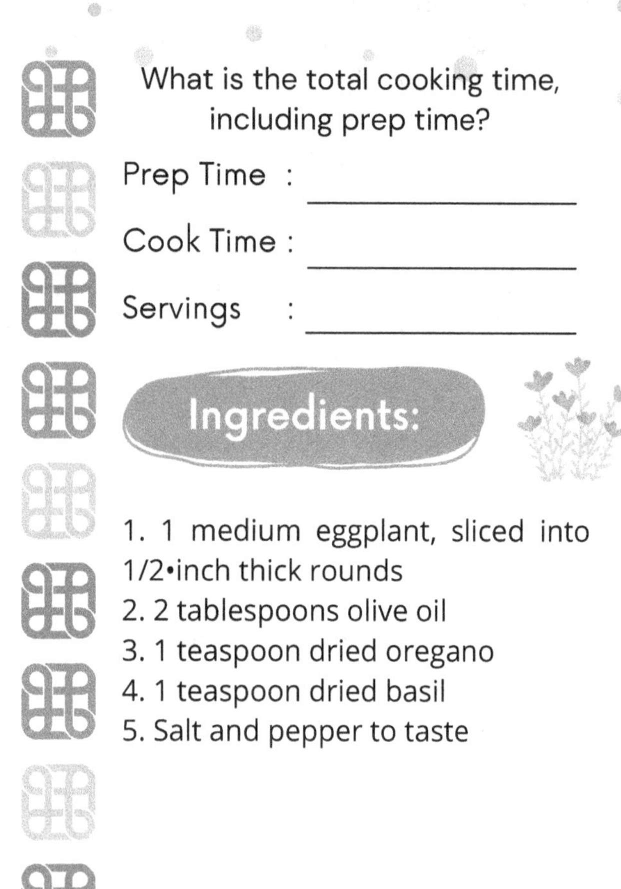

1. 1 medium eggplant, sliced into 1/2•inch thick rounds
2. 2 tablespoons olive oil
3. 1 teaspoon dried oregano
4. 1 teaspoon dried basil
5. Salt and pepper to taste

Is the recipe easy to follow?

33. Grilled eggplant with herbs

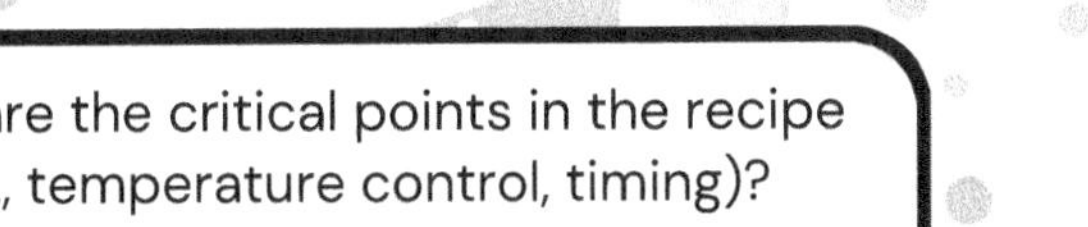 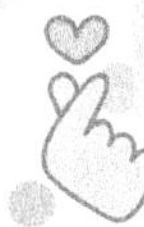

What are the critical points in the recipe (e.g., temperature control, timing)?

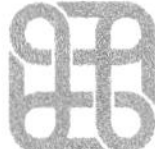 What is the total cooking time, including prep time?

Prep Time : _______________

Cook Time : _______________

Servings   : _______________

Ingredients: 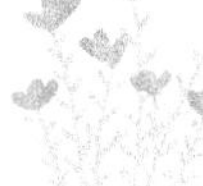

1. 1 medium butternut squash, peeled, seeded, and cubed
2. 2 tablespoons olive oil
3. 1 teaspoon ground cinnamon
4. 1/2 teaspoon ground turmeric
5. Salt and pepper to taste

Is the recipe easy to follow?

34. Baked butternut squash with cinnamon

Procedure:

1. Preheat oven to 400°F (200°C).

2. In a large bowl, toss the cubed butternut squash with the olive oil, cinnamon, turmeric, salt, and pepper until well coated.

3. Spread the seasoned squash cubes in a single layer on a baking sheet lined with parchment paper.

4. Bake for 25•30 minutes, or until the squash is tender and lightly browned, flipping halfway through.

5. Serve the baked butternut squash warm, garnished with extra cinnamon if desired.

The key anti•inflammatory ingredients in this recipe are:

• Butternut squash: Rich in antioxidants and anti•inflammatory nutrients like vitamin A, vitamin C, and carotenoids.
• Cinnamon: Has potent anti•inflammatory properties and can help reduce oxidative stress.
• Turmeric: Contains the active compound curcumin, which is a powerful anti•inflammatory.

This simple, flavorful dish is a great way to enjoy the health benefits of butternut squash and anti•inflammatory spices.

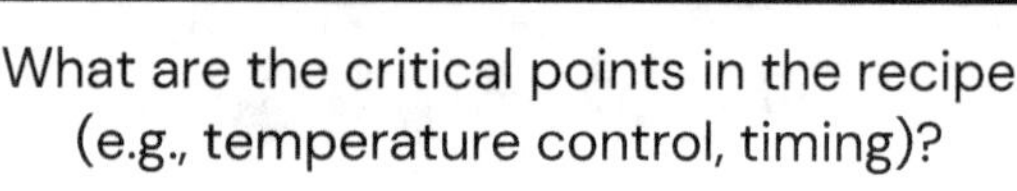
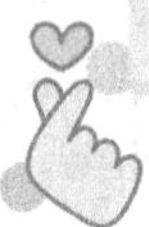

What are the critical points in the recipe (e.g., temperature control, timing)?

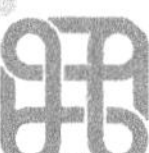

What is the total cooking time, including prep time?

Prep Time : _______________

Cook Time : _______________

Servings   : _______________

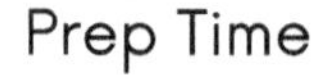

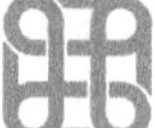
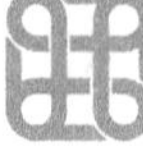

1. 2 cups diced cucumber
2. 1 cup cherry or grape tomatoes, halved
3. 1 tablespoon extra•virgin olive oil
4. 1 tablespoon red wine vinegar
5. 1 teaspoon dried oregano

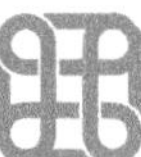
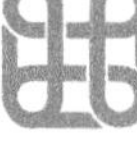
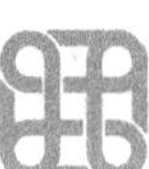
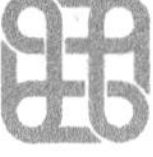
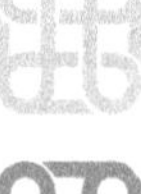
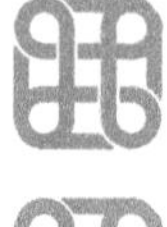
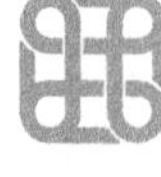
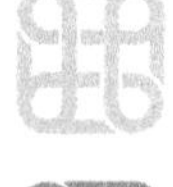
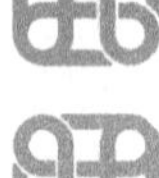
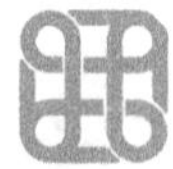

Is the recipe easy to follow?

35. Cucumber and tomato salad

1. In a medium bowl, combine the diced cucumber and halved tomatoes.

2. Drizzle the olive oil and red wine vinegar over the vegetables and toss gently to coat.

3. Sprinkle the dried oregano over the salad and season with salt and pepper to taste.

4. Toss the salad again to evenly distribute the dressing and seasonings.

5. Cover and refrigerate for at least 30 minutes to allow the flavors to meld.

6. Serve chilled or at room temperature.

The key anti•inflammatory ingredients in this recipe are:

• Cucumber: Contains antioxidants and compounds that can help reduce inflammation.
• Tomatoes: Rich in the antioxidant lycopene, which has potent anti•inflammatory properties.
• Olive oil: Contains healthy monounsaturated fats that can help reduce inflammation.
• Oregano: Has strong anti•inflammatory and antioxidant effects.

This refreshing and flavorful salad is a great way to incorporate anti•inflammatory foods into your diet. Enjoy it as a side dish or a light main course.

What are the critical points in the recipe (e.g., temperature control, timing)?

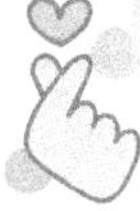

1. Preheat your oven to 400°F (200°C).

2. Pat the drained and rinsed chickpeas dry with a paper towel or clean kitchen towel.

3. In a medium bowl, toss the chickpeas with the olive oil, turmeric, cumin, salt, and pepper until the chickpeas are evenly coated.

4. Spread the seasoned chickpeas in a single layer on a baking sheet lined with parchment paper.

5. Roast the chickpeas for 20·25 minutes, shaking the pan halfway through, until they are crispy and golden brown.

6. Remove the roasted chickpeas from the oven and let them cool for a few minutes before serving.

The key anti·inflammatory ingredients in this recipe are:

• Chickpeas: A good source of fiber, protein, and anti·inflammatory nutrients like folate and magnesium.
• Turmeric: Contains the active compound curcumin, which has potent anti·inflammatory properties.
• Cumin: Has anti·inflammatory and antioxidant effects that can help reduce oxidative stress.

These crispy, flavorful roasted chickpeas make a great snack or addition to salads, bowls, and other dishes. Enjoy the health benefits of this simple, anti·inflammatory recipe.

What is the total cooking time, including prep time?

Prep Time : ______________

Cook Time : ______________

Servings : ______________

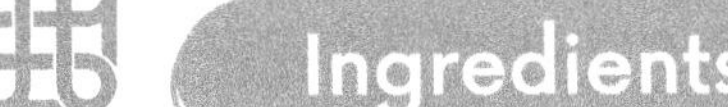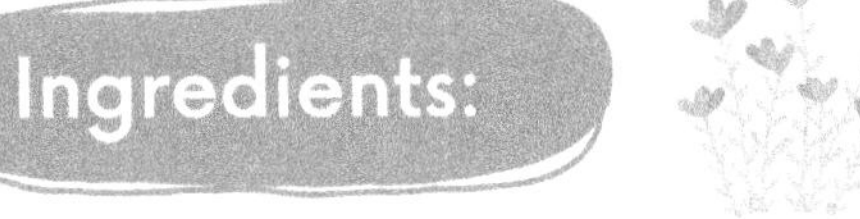
Ingredients:

1. 1 (15 oz) can of chickpeas, drained and rinsed
2. 1 tablespoon olive oil
3. 1 teaspoon ground turmeric
4. 1/2 teaspoon ground cumin
5. Salt and pepper to taste

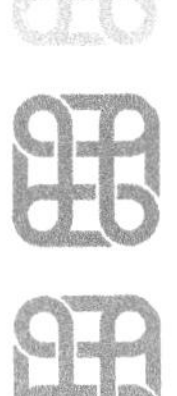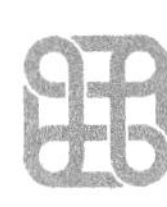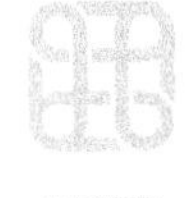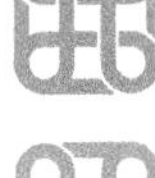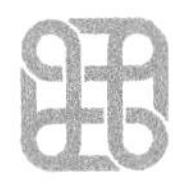

Is the recipe easy to follow?

36. Roasted chickpeas with turmeric

What are the critical points in the recipe (e.g., temperature control, timing)?

What is the total cooking time, including prep time?

Prep Time : _______________

Cook Time : _______________

Servings   : _______________

Ingredients:

1. 4 ripe peaches, halved and pitted
2. 2 tablespoons coconut oil, melted
3. 1 teaspoon ground cinnamon
4. 1 teaspoon ground ginger
5. 1 tablespoon raw honey (optional)

Is the recipe easy to follow?

☺ ☹

37. Grilled peaches with cinnamon

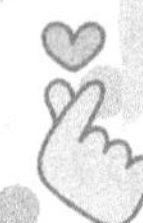

Procedure:

1. Preheat your grill or grill pan to medium•high heat.

2. In a small bowl, combine the melted coconut oil, cinnamon, and ginger. Mix well.

3. Brush the cut side of the peach halves with the cinnamon•ginger oil mixture.

4. Place the peach halves, cut•side down, on the preheated grill. Grill for 3•5 minutes, or until grill marks appear and the peaches are slightly softened.

5. Carefully flip the peach halves and grill for an additional 2•3 minutes, or until they are tender and slightly charred.

6. Remove the grilled peaches from the grill and drizzle with a small amount of raw honey, if desired.

7. Serve the warm, grilled peaches immediately.

The key anti•inflammatory ingredients in this recipe are:

• Peaches: Rich in antioxidants and anti•inflammatory vitamins like vitamin C and vitamin A.
• Cinnamon: Has potent anti•inflammatory properties and can help reduce oxidative stress.
• Ginger: Contains the active compound gingerol, which has strong anti•inflammatory effects.
• Coconut oil: Provides healthy fats that can help reduce inflammation.

This simple, yet delicious grilled peach dessert is a great way to enjoy the health benefits of anti•inflammatory foods.

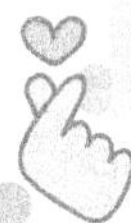

What are the critical points in the recipe (e.g., temperature control, timing)?

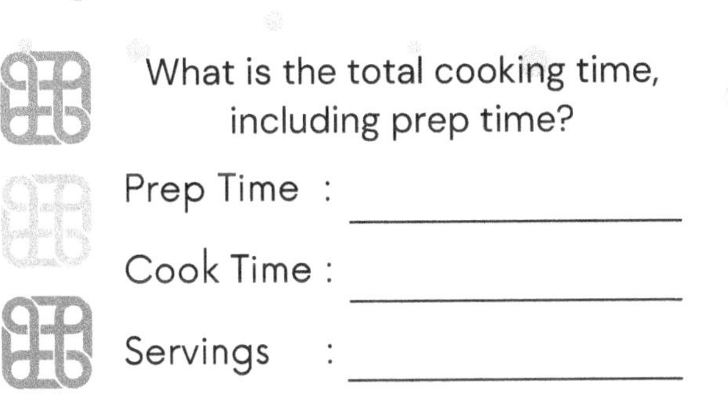

What is the total cooking time, including prep time?

Prep Time : ________________

Cook Time : ________________

Servings   : ________________

Ingredients:

1. 8 oz. cremini or button mushrooms, sliced
2. 2 tablespoons extra•virgin olive oil
3. 3 cloves garlic, minced
4. 1 teaspoon dried thyme
5. Salt and pepper to taste

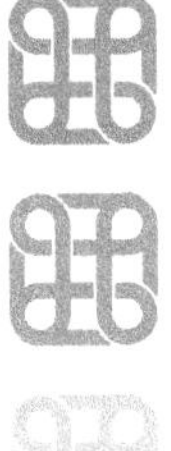
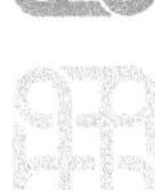
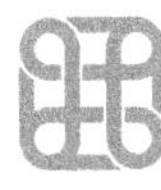
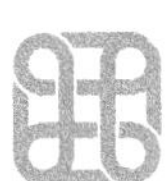

Is the recipe easy to follow?

38. Sautéed mushrooms with garlic

1. In a large skillet, heat the olive oil over medium•high heat.

2. Add the sliced mushrooms to the skillet and sauté for 5•7 minutes, stirring occasionally, until the mushrooms are tender and lightly browned.

3. Add the minced garlic to the skillet and continue cooking for an additional 1•2 minutes, until the garlic is fragrant.

4. Sprinkle the dried thyme over the sautéed mushrooms and garlic, and season with salt and pepper to taste.

5. Stir to combine and cook for another minute or two, until the thyme is fragrant.

6. Remove the skillet from heat and serve the sautéed mushrooms warm.

The key anti•inflammatory ingredients in this recipe are:

• Mushrooms: Contain antioxidants and anti•inflammatory compounds like selenium and ergothioneine.
• Garlic: Has potent anti•inflammatory and antimicrobial properties.
• Olive oil: Provides healthy monounsaturated fats with anti•inflammatory benefits.
• Thyme: Contains the compound thymol, which has strong anti•inflammatory effects.

This simple, flavorful sautéed mushroom dish is a great way to incorporate anti•inflammatory foods into your diet. Enjoy it as a side dish or add it to salads, pasta, or other meals.

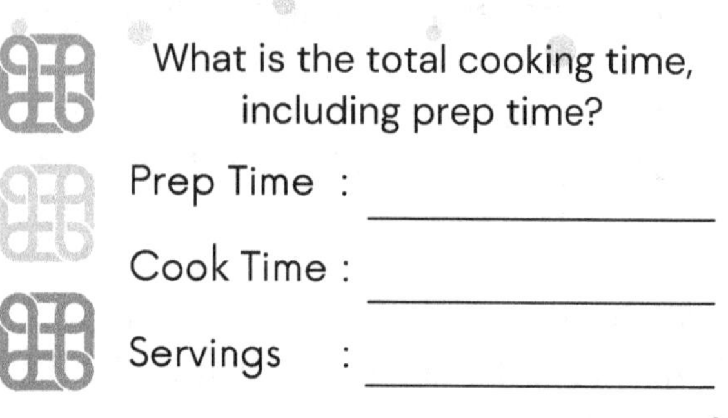

What is the total cooking time,
including prep time?

Prep Time : _______________

Cook Time : _______________

Servings   : _______________

Ingredients:

1. 4 (6 oz) cod fillets
2. 2 tablespoons extra•virgin olive oil
3. 2 tablespoons freshly squeezed lemon juice
4. 2 tablespoons chopped fresh dill
5. Salt and pepper to taste

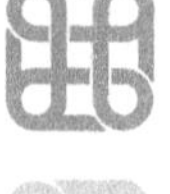
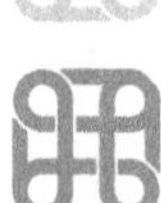
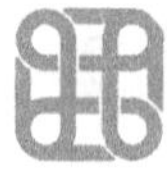

**Is the recipe easy to
follow?**

39. Baked cod with lemon and dill

Procedure:

1. Preheat your oven to 400°F (200°C).

2. Place the cod fillets in a baking dish or on a parchment•lined baking sheet.

3. In a small bowl, whisk together the olive oil, lemon juice, and chopped dill.

4. Drizzle the lemon•dill mixture over the cod fillets, making sure to evenly coat the fish.

5. Season the cod with salt and pepper to taste.

6. Bake the cod for 12•15 minutes, or until it flakes easily with a fork and is opaque throughout.

7. Serve the baked cod immediately, garnished with additional fresh dill if desired.

The key anti•inflammatory ingredients in this recipe are:

• Cod: A lean, protein•rich fish that is low in mercury and high in anti•inflammatory omega•3 fatty acids.
• Lemon: Contains vitamin C and citric acid, which have anti•inflammatory properties.
• Dill: Has potent antioxidant and anti•inflammatory effects.
• Olive oil: Provides healthy monounsaturated fats that can help reduce inflammation.

This simple, flavorful baked cod dish is a great way to enjoy the health benefits of anti•inflammatory foods. Serve it with roasted vegetables or a fresh salad for a complete, nourishing meal.

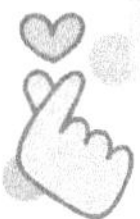

What are the critical points in the recipe (e.g., temperature control, timing)?

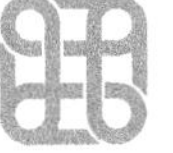 What is the total cooking time, including prep time?

Prep Time : ___________________

Cook Time : ___________________

Servings   : ___________________

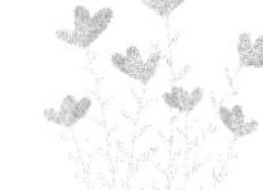
Ingredients:

1. 4 medium beets, peeled and cut into 1•inch cubes
2. 2 tablespoons extra•virgin olive oil
3. 2 tablespoons balsamic vinegar
4. 1 teaspoon dried thyme
5. Salt and pepper to taste

Is the recipe easy to follow?

40. Roasted beets with balsamic vinegar

Procedure:

1. Preheat your oven to 400°F (200°C).

2. In a large bowl, toss the cubed beets with the olive oil, balsamic vinegar, thyme, salt, and pepper until the beets are evenly coated.

3. Spread the seasoned beets in a single layer on a baking sheet lined with parchment paper.

4. Roast the beets for 25•30 minutes, or until they are tender and lightly caramelized, stirring halfway through.

5. Remove the roasted beets from the oven and let them cool for a few minutes before serving.

The key anti•inflammatory ingredients in this recipe are:

• Beets: Rich in antioxidants, vitamins, and anti•inflammatory compounds like betalains.
• Balsamic vinegar: Contains polyphenols that can help reduce inflammation.
• Olive oil: Provides healthy monounsaturated fats with anti•inflammatory properties.
• Thyme: Has strong anti•inflammatory and antioxidant effects.

This simple, flavorful roasted beet dish is a great way to incorporate anti•inflammatory foods into your diet. Enjoy it as a side dish or add it to salads, bowls, or other meals.

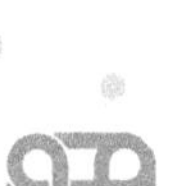
What is the total cooking time, including prep time?

Prep Time : ___________________

Cook Time : ___________________

Servings   : ___________________

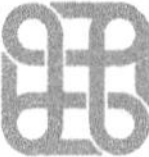
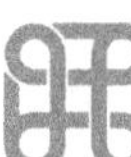
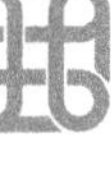
Ingredients:

1. 1 cup plain Greek yogurt
2. 1 cup mixed berries (such as blueberries, raspberries, and/or strawberries)
3. 1 tablespoon ground flaxseed
4. 1 teaspoon honey (optional)
5. Pinch of cinnamon

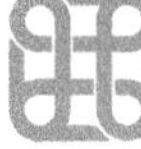
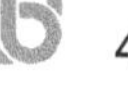
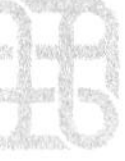
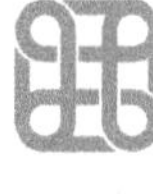
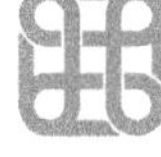
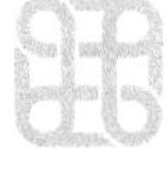
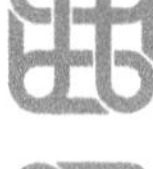
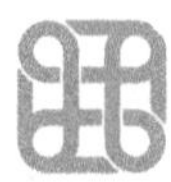

Is the recipe easy to follow?

41. Greek yogurt with berries and flaxseed

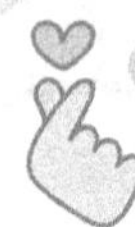
Procedure:

1. In a medium bowl, combine the Greek yogurt and mixed berries.

2. Sprinkle the ground flaxseed over the yogurt and berries.

3. If desired, drizzle the honey over the top.

4. Finish with a light dusting of cinnamon.

5. Gently stir the ingredients together until well combined.

6. Serve immediately or refrigerate until ready to enjoy.

The key anti•inflammatory ingredients in this recipe are:

• Greek yogurt: A good source of protein and probiotics, which can help reduce inflammation.
• Berries: Rich in antioxidants and anti•inflammatory compounds like anthocyanins.
• Flaxseed: Contains anti•inflammatory omega•3 fatty acids and lignans.
• Cinnamon: Has potent anti•inflammatory and antioxidant properties.

This simple, nutrient•dense parfait is a great way to start your day or enjoy as a healthy snack. The combination of creamy yogurt, sweet berries, and anti•inflammatory ingredients makes it a delicious and nourishing option.

What is the total cooking time, including prep time?

Prep Time : ________________

Cook Time : ________________

Servings   : ________________

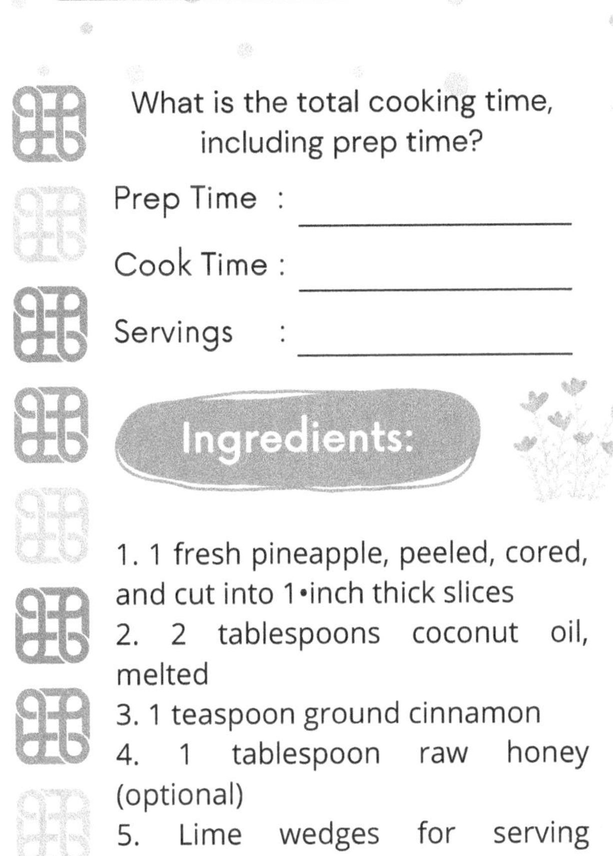

Ingredients:

1. 1 fresh pineapple, peeled, cored, and cut into 1•inch thick slices
2. 2 tablespoons coconut oil, melted
3. 1 teaspoon ground cinnamon
4. 1 tablespoon raw honey (optional)
5. Lime wedges for serving (optional)

Is the recipe easy to follow?

42. Grilled pineapple with cinnamon

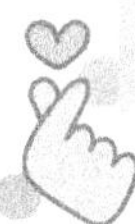

Procedure:

1. Preheat your grill or grill pan to medium•high heat.

2. In a small bowl, combine the melted coconut oil and ground cinnamon. Mix well.

3. Brush the pineapple slices on both sides with the cinnamon•coconut oil mixture.

4. Grill the pineapple slices for 2•3 minutes per side, or until they are lightly charred and softened.

5. Remove the grilled pineapple slices from the grill and drizzle with a small amount of raw honey, if desired.

6. Serve the warm, grilled pineapple slices immediately, with lime wedges on the side if desired.

The key anti•inflammatory ingredients in this recipe are:

• Pineapple: Contains the enzyme bromelain, which has potent anti•inflammatory properties.
• Coconut oil: Provides healthy fats with anti•inflammatory benefits.
• Cinnamon: Has strong anti•inflammatory and antioxidant effects.

This simple, yet delicious grilled pineapple dessert is a great way to enjoy the health benefits of anti•inflammatory foods. The natural sweetness of the pineapple pairs perfectly with the warmth of the cinnamon and coconut oil.

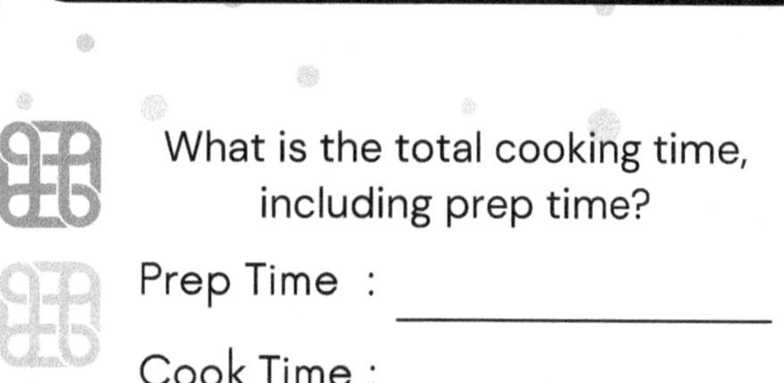

What is the total cooking time, including prep time?

Prep Time : _______________

Cook Time : _______________

Servings   : _______________

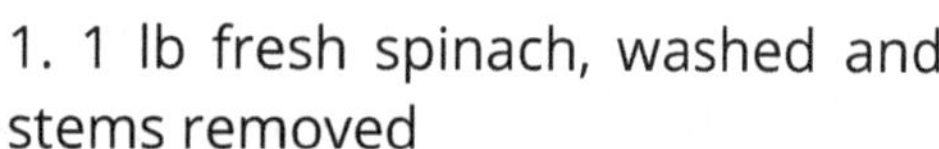

Ingredients:

1. 1 lb fresh spinach, washed and stems removed
2. 2 tablespoons extra•virgin olive oil
3. 3 cloves garlic, minced
4. 1 teaspoon lemon juice
5. Salt and pepper to taste

Is the recipe easy to follow?

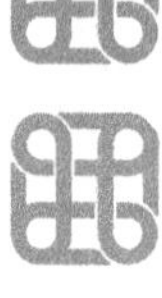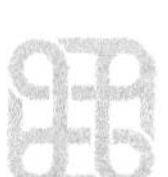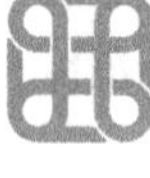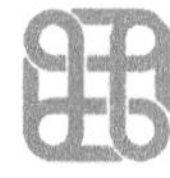

43. Sautéed spinach with garlic

Procedure:

1. In a large skillet or wok, heat the olive oil over medium heat.

2. Add the minced garlic to the hot oil and sauté for 1•2 minutes, until fragrant.

3. Add the fresh spinach to the skillet in batches, if needed, and sauté for 2•3 minutes, stirring frequently, until the spinach is wilted and tender.

4. Drizzle the lemon juice over the sautéed spinach and garlic, and season with salt and pepper to taste.

5. Toss the spinach to evenly distribute the lemon juice and seasonings.

6. Serve the sautéed spinach with garlic warm.

The key anti•inflammatory ingredients in this recipe are:

• Spinach: Rich in antioxidants, vitamins, and anti•inflammatory compounds like lutein and zeaxanthin.
• Garlic: Has potent anti•inflammatory and antimicrobial properties.
• Olive oil: Provides healthy monounsaturated fats with anti•inflammatory benefits.
• Lemon juice: Contains vitamin C and citric acid, which have anti•inflammatory effects.

This simple, flavorful sautéed spinach dish is a great way to incorporate anti•inflammatory foods into your diet. Enjoy it as a side dish or add it to salads, pasta, or other meals.

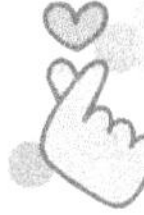

What is the total cooking time, including prep time?

Prep Time : _______________

Cook Time : _______________

Servings : _______________

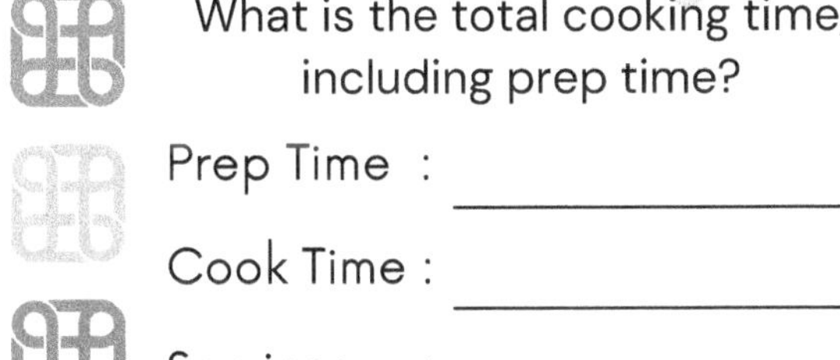

Ingredients:

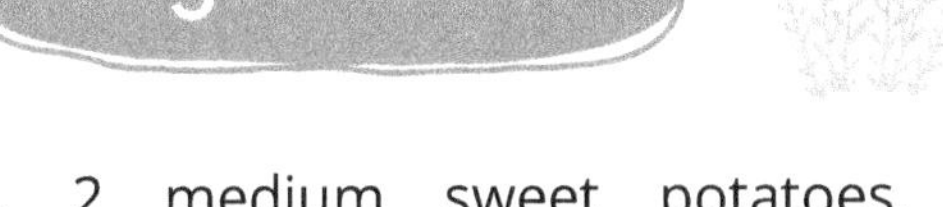

1. 2 medium sweet potatoes, scrubbed and pierced with a fork
2. 1 (15 oz) can of black beans, drained and rinsed
3. 1 tablespoon extra•virgin olive oil
4. 1 teaspoon ground cumin
5. Salt and pepper to taste

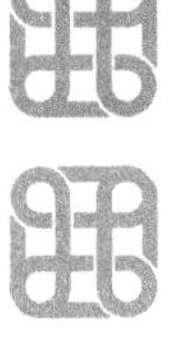
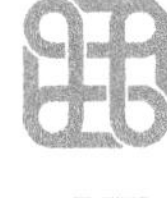
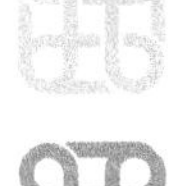
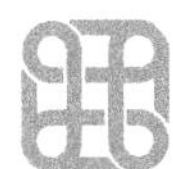

Is the recipe easy to follow?

44. Baked sweet potato with black beans

1. Preheat your oven to 400°F (200°C).

2. Place the pierced sweet potatoes directly on the oven rack and bake for 45•60 minutes, or until they are tender when pierced with a fork.

3. In a small saucepan, combine the drained and rinsed black beans, olive oil, and cumin. Heat over medium heat, stirring occasionally, until the beans are warmed through.

4. Remove the baked sweet potatoes from the oven and let them cool for a few minutes.

5. Slice the sweet potatoes open and top with the warm black bean mixture.

6. Season with salt and pepper to taste.

The key anti•inflammatory ingredients in this recipe are:

• Sweet potatoes: Rich in anti•inflammatory antioxidants like beta•carotene and vitamin C.
• Black beans: A good source of fiber, protein, and anti•inflammatory polyphenols.
• Olive oil: Provides healthy monounsaturated fats with anti•inflammatory benefits.
• Cumin: Has potent anti•inflammatory and antioxidant properties.

This simple, nutrient•dense baked sweet potato and black bean dish is a great way to enjoy the health benefits of anti•inflammatory foods. Serve it as a main course or a side dish.

What are the critical points in the recipe (e.g., temperature control, timing)?

What is the total cooking time, including prep time?

Prep Time : _______________

Cook Time : _______________

Servings   : _______________

1. 1 pint cherry or grape tomatoes, halved
2. 2 tablespoons extra•virgin olive oil
3. 2 cloves garlic, minced
4. 1/4 cup fresh basil leaves, chopped
5. Salt and pepper to taste

Is the recipe easy to follow?

45. Roasted cherry tomatoes with basil

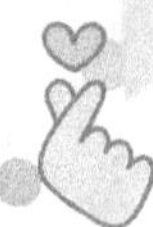

1. Preheat your oven to 400°F (200°C).

2. In a large bowl, toss the halved cherry tomatoes with the olive oil, minced garlic, salt, and pepper until the tomatoes are evenly coated.

3. Spread the seasoned tomatoes in a single layer on a baking sheet lined with parchment paper.

4. Roast the tomatoes for 15•20 minutes, or until they are softened and starting to burst.

5. Remove the roasted tomatoes from the oven and transfer them to a serving bowl.

6. Sprinkle the chopped fresh basil over the roasted tomatoes and gently toss to combine.

7. Serve the roasted cherry tomatoes with basil warm or at room temperature.

The key anti•inflammatory ingredients in this recipe are:

• Cherry tomatoes: Rich in the antioxidant lycopene, which has potent anti•inflammatory properties.
• Olive oil: Provides healthy monounsaturated fats with anti•inflammatory benefits.
• Garlic: Has strong anti•inflammatory and antimicrobial effects.
• Basil: Contains compounds like eugenol and citronellol that have anti•inflammatory effects.

This simple, flavorful roasted tomato dish is a great way to enjoy the health benefits of anti•inflammatory foods. Serve it as a side dish or use it to top salads, pasta, or other meals.

What are the critical points in the recipe (e.g., temperature control, timing)?

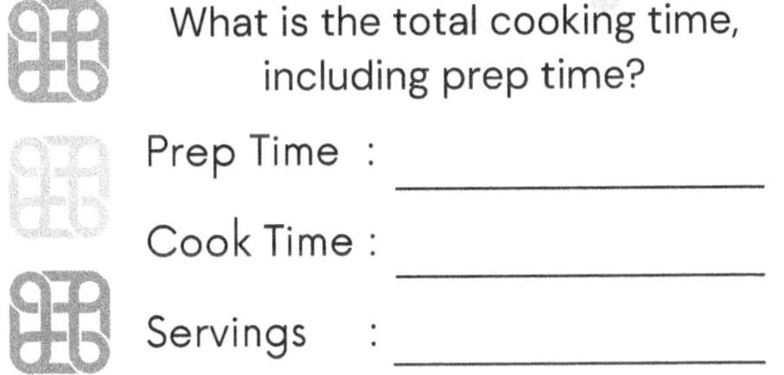

What is the total cooking time, including prep time?

Prep Time : _______________

Cook Time : _______________

Servings   : _______________

Ingredients:

1. 1 lb fresh asparagus, trimmed
2. 2 tablespoons extra·virgin olive oil
3. 1 tablespoon freshly squeezed lemon juice
4. 1 teaspoon grated lemon zest
5. Salt and pepper to taste

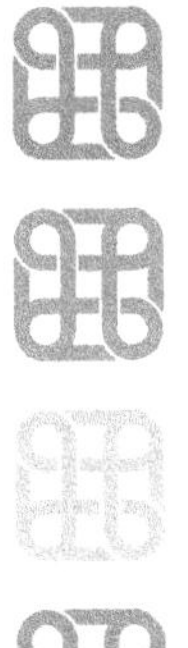

Is the recipe easy to follow?

46. Grilled asparagus with lemon

1. Preheat your grill or grill pan to medium·high heat.

2. In a large bowl, toss the trimmed asparagus spears with the olive oil, lemon juice, and a pinch of salt and pepper.

3. Arrange the seasoned asparagus in a single layer on the preheated grill or grill pan.

4. Grill the asparagus for 3·5 minutes per side, or until they are tender and lightly charred.

5. Transfer the grilled asparagus to a serving plate and sprinkle the grated lemon zest over the top.

6. Serve the warm, grilled asparagus immediately.

The key anti·inflammatory ingredients in this recipe are:

• Asparagus: Rich in antioxidants, vitamins, and anti·inflammatory compounds like glutathione and rutin.
• Olive oil: Provides healthy monounsaturated fats with anti·inflammatory benefits.
• Lemon: Contains vitamin C and citric acid, which have anti·inflammatory properties.

This simple, flavorful grilled asparagus dish is a great way to enjoy the health benefits of anti·inflammatory foods. Serve it as a side dish or add it to salads, bowls, or other meals.

Procedure:

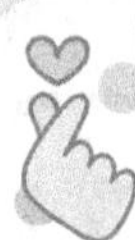

1. Preheat your oven to 200°F (95°C).

2. Line two baking sheets with parchment paper.

3. In a small bowl, combine the melted coconut oil, cinnamon, and a pinch of salt. Mix well.

4. Arrange the apple slices in a single layer on the prepared baking sheets. Brush or drizzle the cinnamon•coconut oil mixture over the apple slices, making sure to coat both sides.

5. Bake the apple chips for 2•3 hours, flipping them halfway through, until they are crispy and lightly browned.

6. Remove the baked apple chips from the oven and let them cool completely.

7. If desired, drizzle the cooled apple chips with a small amount of raw honey.

The key anti•inflammatory ingredients in this recipe are:

• Apples: Rich in antioxidants and anti•inflammatory compounds like quercetin and flavonoids.
• Coconut oil: Provides healthy fats with anti•inflammatory benefits.
• Cinnamon: Has potent anti•inflammatory and antioxidant properties.
• Honey (optional): Contains anti•inflammatory and antimicrobial properties.

These crispy, flavorful baked apple chips make a great healthy snack or topping for yogurt, oatmeal, or other dishes. Enjoy the anti•inflammatory benefits of this simple recipe.

What is the total cooking time, including prep time?

Prep Time : ________________

Cook Time : ________________

Servings   : ________________

Ingredients:

1. 2 medium apples, thinly sliced (about 1/8•inch thick)
2. 1 tablespoon coconut oil, melted
3. 1 teaspoon ground cinnamon
4. 1 tablespoon raw honey (optional)
5. Pinch of salt

Is the recipe easy to follow?

47. Baked apple chips with cinnamon

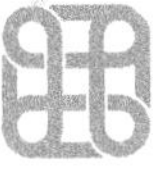

What is the total cooking time, including prep time?

Prep Time : _________________

Cook Time : _________________

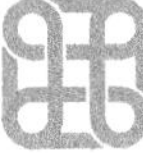

Servings : _________________

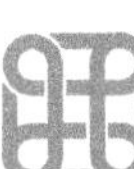
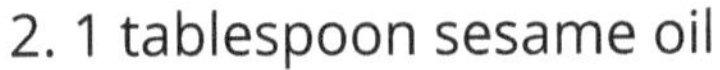

Ingredients:

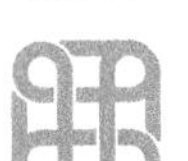
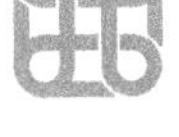

1. 1 lb bok choy, stems and leaves separated and chopped
2. 1 tablespoon sesame oil
3. 2 teaspoons freshly grated ginger
4. 1 tablespoon low·sodium soy sauce or tamari
5. Salt and pepper to taste

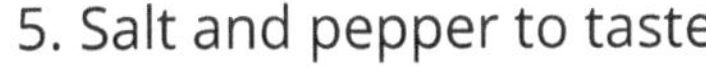
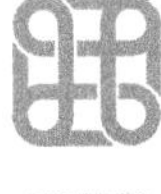
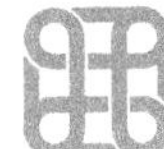

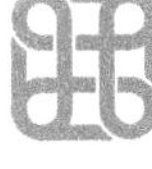
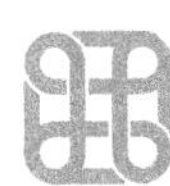

Is the recipe easy to follow?

48. Sautéed bok choy with ginger

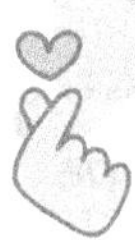

Procedure:

1. In a large skillet or wok, heat the sesame oil over medium·high heat.

2. Add the chopped bok choy stems to the skillet and sauté for 2·3 minutes, until they start to soften.

3. Add the chopped bok choy leaves and the grated ginger to the skillet. Sauté for an additional 2·3 minutes, stirring frequently, until the leaves are wilted and tender.

4. Drizzle the soy sauce or tamari over the sautéed bok choy and ginger, and toss to coat evenly.

5. Season the dish with salt and pepper to taste.

6. Serve the sautéed bok choy with ginger warm.

The key anti·inflammatory ingredients in this recipe are:

• Bok choy: A cruciferous vegetable rich in antioxidants and anti·inflammatory compounds like vitamin K and sulforaphane.
• Ginger: Contains the active compound gingerol, which has potent anti·inflammatory properties.
• Sesame oil: Provides healthy fats with anti·inflammatory benefits.
• Soy sauce or tamari: Contains anti·inflammatory compounds like isoflavones.

This simple, flavorful sautéed bok choy dish is a great way to incorporate anti·inflammatory foods into your diet. Serve it as a side dish or add it to stir·fries, bowls, or other meals.

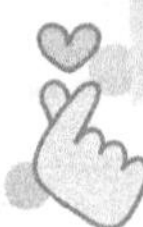

Procedure:

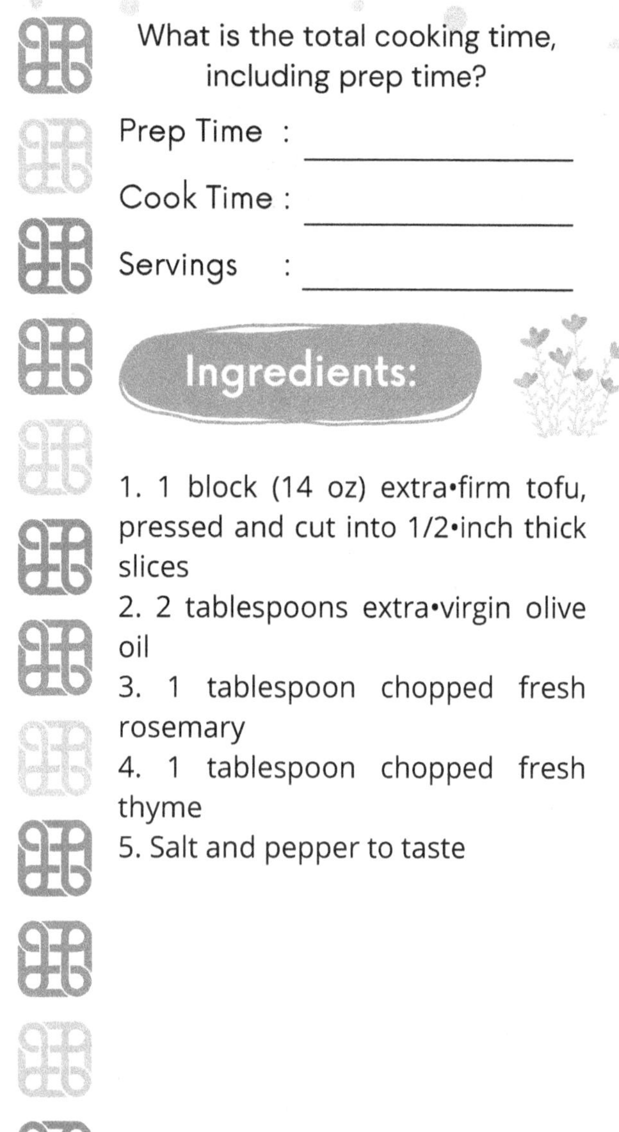

What is the total cooking time, including prep time?

Prep Time : _______________

Cook Time : _______________

Servings : _______________

Ingredients:

1. 1 block (14 oz) extra•firm tofu, pressed and cut into 1/2•inch thick slices
2. 2 tablespoons extra•virgin olive oil
3. 1 tablespoon chopped fresh rosemary
4. 1 tablespoon chopped fresh thyme
5. Salt and pepper to taste

Is the recipe easy to follow?

49. Grilled tofu with herbs

1. Preheat your grill or grill pan to medium•high heat.

2. In a shallow dish, combine the olive oil, chopped rosemary, and chopped thyme. Add the tofu slices and gently toss to coat them evenly with the herb•infused oil.

3. Season the tofu slices with salt and pepper.

4. Carefully place the tofu slices on the preheated grill or grill pan. Grill for 3•4 minutes per side, or until they are lightly charred and have grill marks.

5. Remove the grilled tofu from the heat and transfer it to a serving plate.

6. Serve the warm, grilled tofu immediately, garnished with any remaining fresh herbs if desired.

The key anti•inflammatory ingredients in this recipe are:

• Tofu: A plant•based protein source that is low in saturated fat and high in anti•inflammatory isoflavones.
• Olive oil: Provides healthy monounsaturated fats with anti•inflammatory benefits.
• Rosemary: Contains anti•inflammatory compounds like carnosic acid and rosmarinic acid.
• Thyme: Has strong anti•inflammatory and antioxidant properties.

This simple, flavorful grilled tofu dish is a great way to incorporate anti•inflammatory foods into your diet. Serve it as a main course or add it to salads, bowls, or other meals.

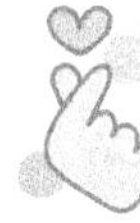

1. Preheat your oven to 400°F (200°C).

2. In a large bowl, toss the trimmed and halved/quartered radishes with the olive oil, dried thyme, Dijon mustard, salt, and pepper until the radishes are evenly coated.

3. Spread the seasoned radishes in a single layer on a baking sheet lined with parchment paper.

4. Roast the radishes for 20•25 minutes, stirring halfway, until they are tender and lightly browned.

5. Remove the roasted radishes from the oven and serve them warm.

The key anti•inflammatory ingredients in this recipe are:

•　Radishes: Contain anti•inflammatory compounds like vitamin C, anthocyanins, and isothiocyanates.
• Olive oil: Provides healthy monounsaturated fats with anti•inflammatory benefits.
• Thyme: Has strong anti•inflammatory and antioxidant properties.
• Dijon mustard: Contains compounds that can help reduce inflammation.

This simple, flavorful roasted radish dish is a great way to incorporate anti•inflammatory foods into your diet. Enjoy it as a side dish or add it to salads, bowls, or other meals.

What is the total cooking time, including prep time?

Prep Time　:　________________

Cook Time :　________________

Servings　　:　________________

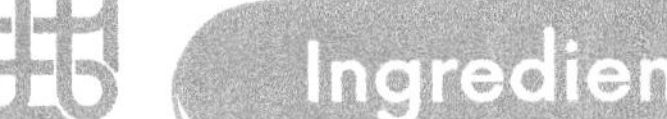

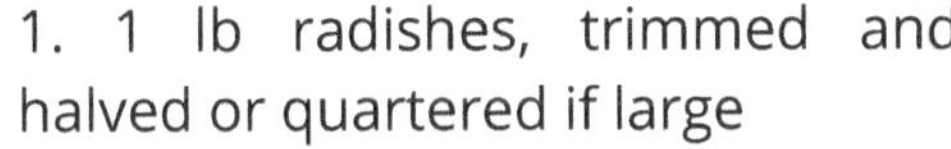

1. 1 lb radishes, trimmed and halved or quartered if large
2. 2 tablespoons extra•virgin olive oil
3. 1 teaspoon dried thyme
4. 1 teaspoon Dijon mustard
5. Salt and pepper to taste

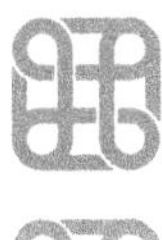
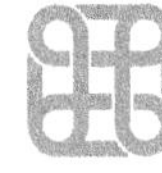
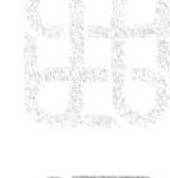
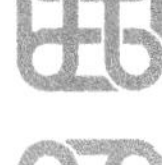
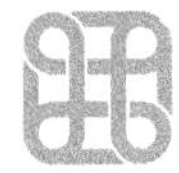

Is the recipe easy to follow?

50. Roasted radishes with olive oil

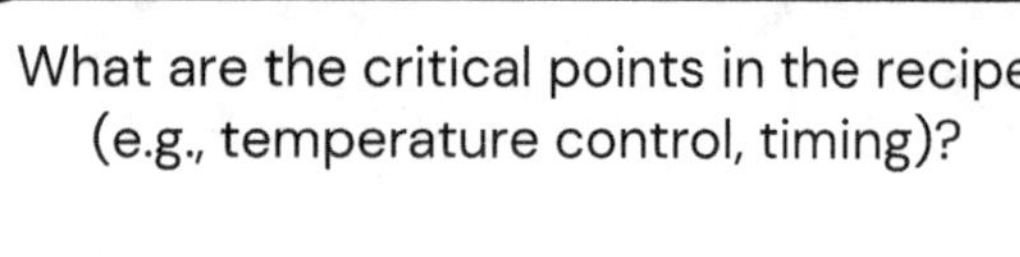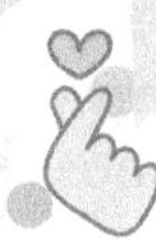

What are the critical points in the recipe (e.g., temperature control, timing)?

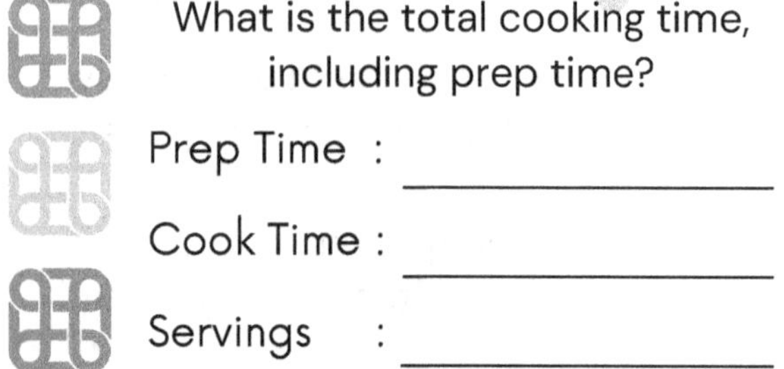

What is the total cooking time, including prep time?

Prep Time : _______________

Cook Time : _______________

Servings : _______________

Ingredients:

1. 2 ripe pears, halved and cored
2. 2 tablespoons raw honey
3. 2 tablespoons chopped walnuts
4. 1 teaspoon ground cinnamon
5. 1 tablespoon coconut oil, melted

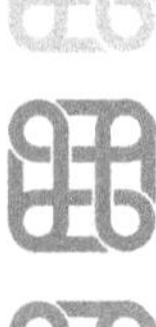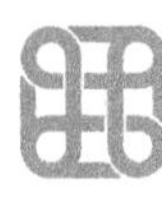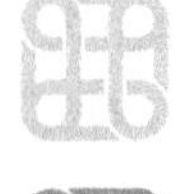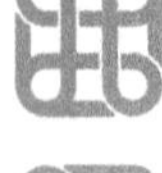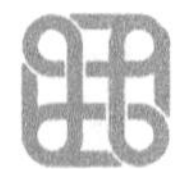

Is the recipe easy to follow?

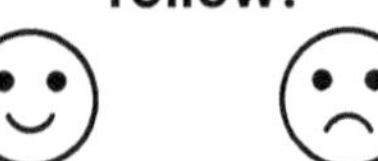

51. Baked pear with walnuts

1. Preheat your oven to 375°F (190°C).

2. Place the pear halves, cut•side up, in a baking dish.

3. In a small bowl, mix together the honey, chopped walnuts, and cinnamon.

4. Spoon the honey•walnut mixture evenly into the cored centers of the pear halves.

5. Drizzle the melted coconut oil over the top of the stuffed pears.

6. Bake the pears for 20•25 minutes, or until they are tender and the topping is lightly browned.

7. Serve the baked pears warm.

The key anti•inflammatory ingredients in this recipe are:

• Pears: Rich in antioxidants and anti•inflammatory compounds like vitamin C and flavonoids.
• Walnuts: Contain anti•inflammatory omega•3 fatty acids and polyphenols.
• Cinnamon: Has potent anti•inflammatory and antioxidant properties.
• Coconut oil: Provides healthy fats with anti•inflammatory benefits.

This simple, yet delicious baked pear dessert is a great way to enjoy the health benefits of anti•inflammatory foods. The natural sweetness of the pear pairs perfectly with the crunch of the walnuts and the warmth of the cinnamon.

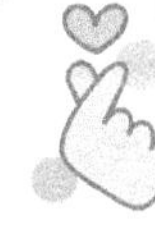

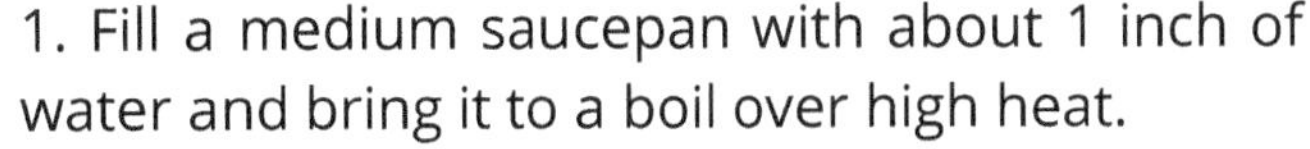

What are the critical points in the recipe (e.g., temperature control, timing)?

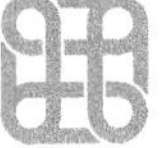

What is the total cooking time, including prep time?

Prep Time : _______________

Cook Time : _______________

Servings   : _______________

Ingredients:

1. 1 lb fresh green beans, trimmed
2. 1 tablespoon extra•virgin olive oil
3. 2 tablespoons sliced almonds
4. 1 teaspoon lemon zest
5. Salt and pepper to taste

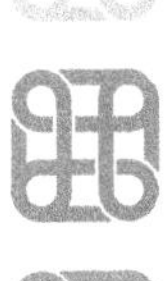
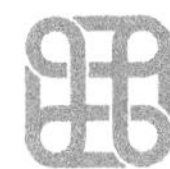
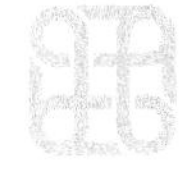
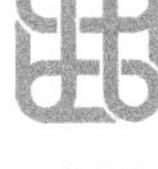
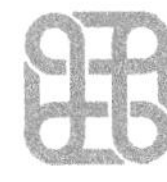

Is the recipe easy to follow?

52. Steamed green beans with almonds

1. Fill a medium saucepan with about 1 inch of water and bring it to a boil over high heat.

2. Add the trimmed green beans to the saucepan, cover, and steam for 5•7 minutes, or until the beans are tender•crisp.

3. Drain the steamed green beans and transfer them to a serving bowl.

4. Drizzle the olive oil over the hot green beans and toss to coat.

5. Sprinkle the sliced almonds and lemon zest over the green beans, and season with salt and pepper to taste.

6. Serve the steamed green beans with almonds warm.

The key anti•inflammatory ingredients in this recipe are:

• Green beans: Rich in antioxidants and anti•inflammatory compounds like vitamin C, vitamin K, and flavonoids.
• Olive oil: Provides healthy monounsaturated fats with anti•inflammatory benefits.
• Almonds: Contain anti•inflammatory healthy fats, vitamin E, and magnesium.
• Lemon zest: Contains vitamin C and citric acid, which have anti•inflammatory properties.

This simple, flavorful steamed green bean dish is a great way to enjoy the health benefits of anti•inflammatory foods. Serve it as a side dish or add it to salads, bowls, or other meals.

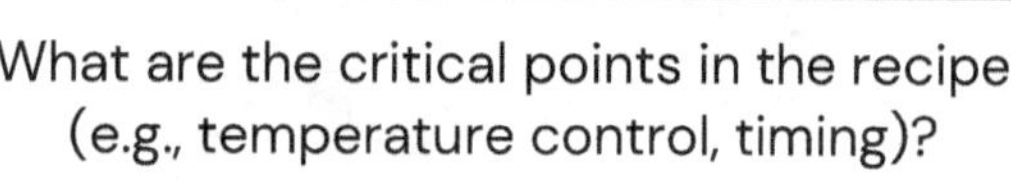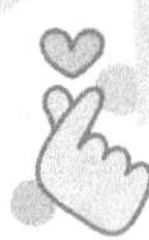

Procedure:

What is the total cooking time, including prep time?

Prep Time : ______________

Cook Time : ______________

Servings : ______________

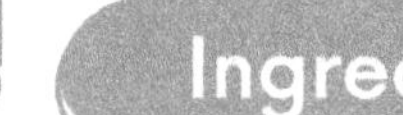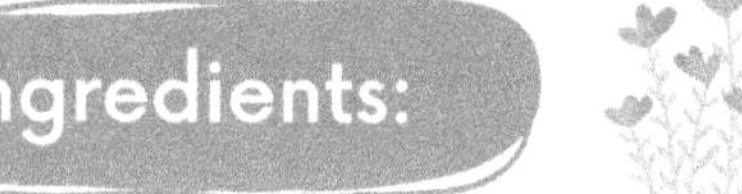

Ingredients:

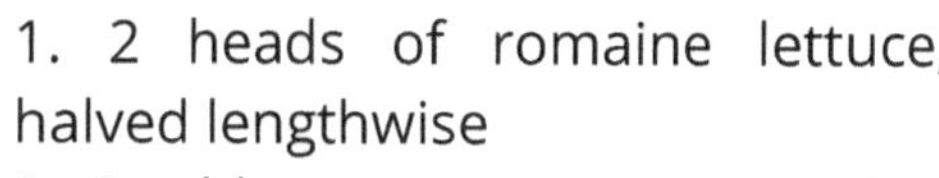

1. 2 heads of romaine lettuce, halved lengthwise
2. 2 tablespoons extra•virgin olive oil
3. Salt and pepper to taste

1. Preheat your grill or grill pan to medium•high heat.

2. Brush the cut sides of the romaine halves with the olive oil, making sure to coat them evenly.

3. Season the oiled romaine halves with salt and pepper.

4. Place the romaine halves, cut•side down, on the preheated grill or grill pan.

5. Grill the romaine for 2•3 minutes per side, or until it's lightly charred and slightly wilted.

6. Remove the grilled romaine from the heat and transfer it to a serving platter.

7. Serve the warm, grilled romaine immediately, drizzling any remaining olive oil over the top if desired.

This simple grilled romaine dish is a great way to add a smoky, charred flavor to your greens. The olive oil helps to keep the romaine from drying out on the grill, and the high heat creates a nice caramelized edge.

You can serve the grilled romaine as a side dish, or use it as the base for a salad with your favorite toppings. It's a quick and easy way to add some variety to your leafy green routine.

Is the recipe easy to follow?

53. Grilled romaine with olive oil

What are the critical points in the recipe (e.g., temperature control, timing)?

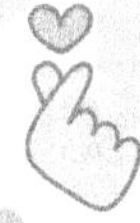

What is the total cooking time, including prep time?

Prep Time : ________________

Cook Time : ________________

Servings   : ________________

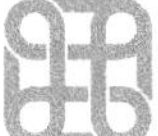

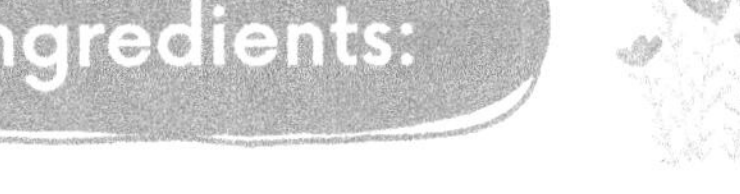
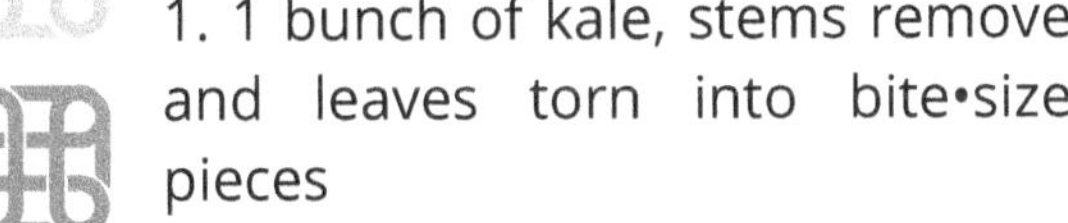

1. 1 bunch of kale, stems removed and leaves torn into bite•sized pieces
2. 1 tablespoon extra•virgin olive oil
3. 2 tablespoons nutritional yeast
4. 1 teaspoon garlic powder
5. Salt and pepper to taste

1. Preheat your oven to 350°F (175°C).

2. In a large bowl, toss the kale leaves with the olive oil, nutritional yeast, garlic powder, salt, and pepper until the kale is evenly coated.

3. Spread the seasoned kale leaves in a single layer on two baking sheets lined with parchment paper.

4. Bake for 12•15 minutes, flipping the kale chips halfway through, until they are crispy and lightly browned.

5. Remove the baked kale chips from the oven and let them cool for a few minutes before serving.

The key anti•inflammatory ingredients in this recipe are:

• Kale: A nutrient•dense leafy green that is rich in antioxidants and anti•inflammatory compounds like vitamin C, vitamin K, and carotenoids.
• Olive oil: Provides healthy monounsaturated fats with anti•inflammatory benefits.
• Nutritional yeast: Contains anti•inflammatory B•vitamins and antioxidants.
• Garlic powder: Has strong anti•inflammatory and antimicrobial properties.

These crispy, flavorful baked kale chips make a great healthy snack or side dish. Enjoy the anti•inflammatory benefits of this simple recipe.

Is the recipe easy to follow?

54. Baked kale chips with nutritional yeast

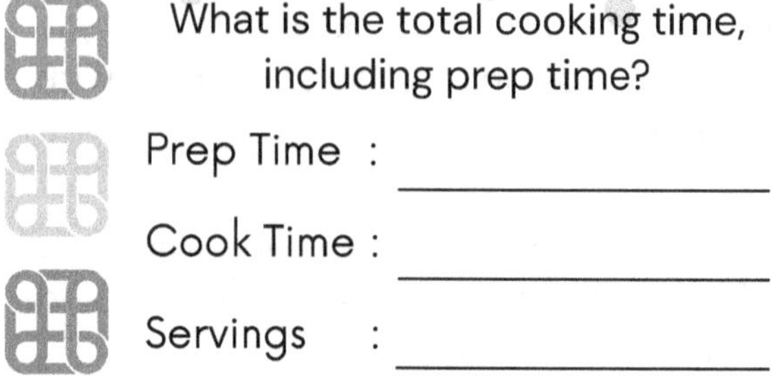

What is the total cooking time, including prep time?

Prep Time : ________________

Cook Time : ________________

Servings   : ________________

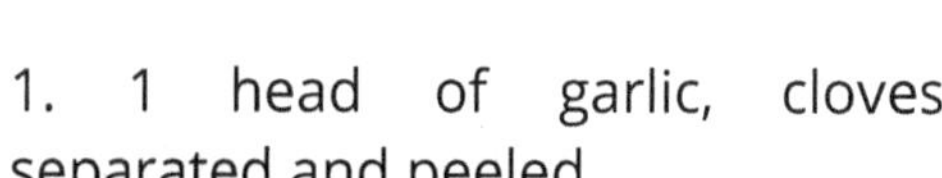

Ingredients:

1. 1 head of garlic, cloves separated and peeled
2. 2 tablespoons extra•virgin olive oil
3. 1 teaspoon dried thyme
4. 1/2 teaspoon ground black pepper
5. Salt to taste

Is the recipe easy to follow?

55. Roasted garlic cloves

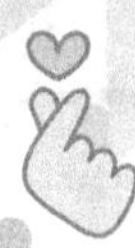

Procedure:

1. Preheat your oven to 400°F (200°C).

2. In a small baking dish or on a baking sheet, toss the peeled garlic cloves with the olive oil, thyme, black pepper, and a pinch of salt.

3. Roast the garlic cloves for 20•25 minutes, stirring halfway, until they are soft, golden brown, and fragrant.

4. Remove the roasted garlic cloves from the oven and let them cool slightly.

5. Serve the roasted garlic cloves warm, either on their own or as a spread on crusty bread or crackers.

The key anti•inflammatory ingredients in this recipe are:

• Garlic: Contains the active compound allicin, which has potent anti•inflammatory and antimicrobial properties.
• Olive oil: Provides healthy monounsaturated fats with anti•inflammatory benefits.
• Thyme: Has strong anti•inflammatory and antioxidant effects.

Roasting the garlic cloves brings out their natural sweetness and mellows their pungent flavor, making them a delicious and versatile anti•inflammatory ingredient. Enjoy these roasted garlic cloves on their own or use them to add flavor to a variety of dishes.

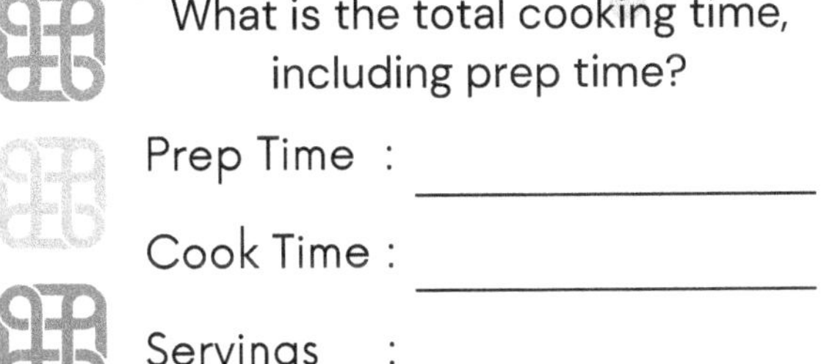

What is the total cooking time, including prep time?

Prep Time : ________________

Cook Time : ________________

Servings   : ________________

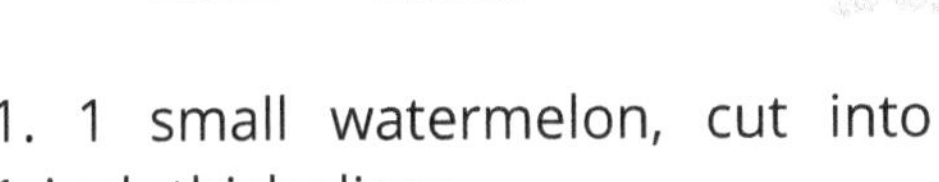

Ingredients:

1. 1 small watermelon, cut into 1•inch thick slices
2. 2 tablespoons extra•virgin olive oil
3. 1 tablespoon balsamic glaze
4. 1/4 cup fresh mint leaves, chopped
5. Pinch of sea salt

Is the recipe easy to follow?

56. Grilled watermelon with mint

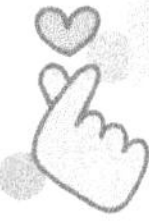

Procedure:

1. Preheat your grill or grill pan to medium•high heat.

2. Brush the watermelon slices on both sides with the olive oil.

3. Grill the watermelon slices for 2•3 minutes per side, or until they have nice grill marks and are slightly softened.

4. Transfer the grilled watermelon slices to a serving platter.

5. Drizzle the balsamic glaze over the grilled watermelon.

6. Sprinkle the chopped fresh mint leaves and a pinch of sea salt over the top.

7. Serve the grilled watermelon with mint immediately, while still warm.

The key anti•inflammatory ingredients in this recipe are:

• Watermelon: Rich in the antioxidant lycopene, which has potent anti•inflammatory properties.
• Olive oil: Provides healthy monounsaturated fats with anti•inflammatory benefits.
• Balsamic glaze: Contains polyphenols that can help reduce inflammation.
• Mint: Has strong anti•inflammatory and antioxidant effects.

This simple, refreshing grilled watermelon dish is a great way to enjoy the health benefits of anti•inflammatory foods. The sweet and savory flavors pair perfectly together, making it a delicious and nourishing summer treat.

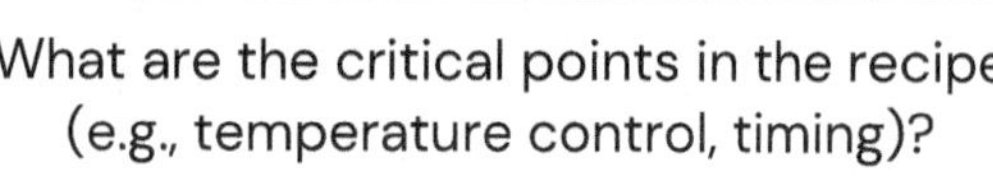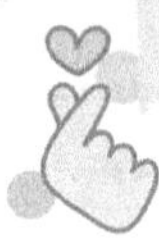

What are the critical points in the recipe (e.g., temperature control, timing)?

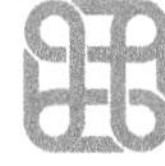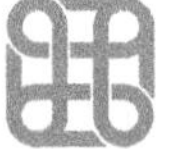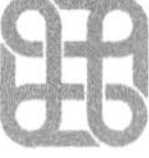 What is the total cooking time, including prep time?

Prep Time : _______________

Cook Time : _______________

Servings : _______________

Ingredients:

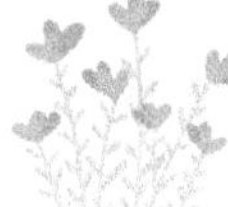

1. 2 medium zucchini, sliced into 1/8•inch thick rounds
2. 1 tablespoon extra•virgin olive oil
3. 1 teaspoon ground turmeric
4. 1/2 teaspoon garlic powder
5. Salt and pepper to taste

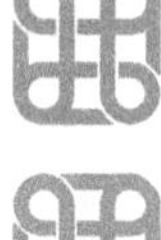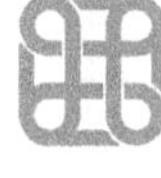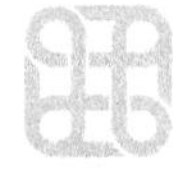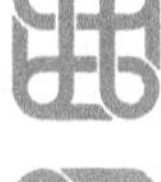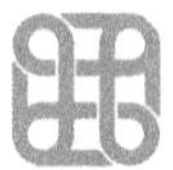

Is the recipe easy to follow?

57. Baked zucchini chips

1. Preheat your oven to 400°F (200°C).

2. Line two baking sheets with parchment paper.

3. In a large bowl, toss the zucchini slices with the olive oil, turmeric, garlic powder, salt, and pepper until the zucchini is evenly coated.

4. Arrange the seasoned zucchini slices in a single layer on the prepared baking sheets, making sure they are not overlapping.

5. Bake for 15•20 minutes, flipping the zucchini chips halfway through, until they are crispy and lightly browned.

6. Remove the baked zucchini chips from the oven and let them cool for a few minutes before serving.

The key anti•inflammatory ingredients in this recipe are:

• Zucchini: Contains antioxidants and anti•inflammatory compounds like vitamin C and carotenoids.
• Olive oil: Provides healthy monounsaturated fats with anti•inflammatory benefits.
• Turmeric: Contains the active compound curcumin, which has potent anti•inflammatory properties.
• Garlic powder: Has strong anti•inflammatory and antimicrobial effects.

These crispy, flavorful baked zucchini chips make a great healthy snack or side dish. Enjoy the anti•inflammatory benefits of this simple recipe.

What is the total cooking time, including prep time?

Prep Time : _______________

Cook Time : _______________

Servings   : _______________

Ingredients:

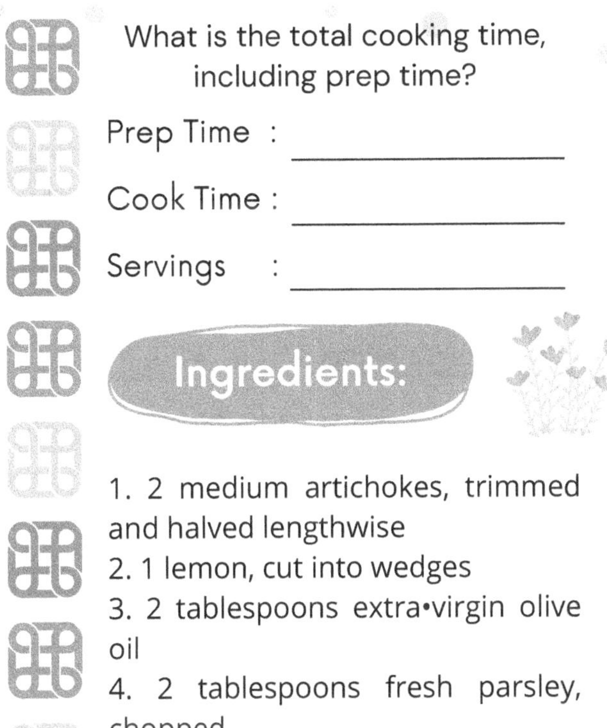

1. 2 medium artichokes, trimmed and halved lengthwise
2. 1 lemon, cut into wedges
3. 2 tablespoons extra•virgin olive oil
4. 2 tablespoons fresh parsley, chopped
5. Salt and pepper to taste

Is the recipe easy to follow?

58. Steamed artichokes with lemon

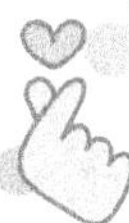

Procedure:

1. Fill a large pot with about 1 inch of water and bring it to a boil over high heat.

2. Place the artichoke halves in a steamer basket and carefully lower it into the boiling water. Cover the pot and steam the artichokes for 20•25 minutes, or until the leaves pull away easily.

3. Remove the steamed artichokes from the pot and transfer them to a serving platter.

4. Drizzle the olive oil over the hot artichokes and squeeze the lemon wedges over the top, allowing the juice to run over the artichokes.

5. Sprinkle the chopped fresh parsley over the artichokes and season with salt and pepper to taste.

6. Serve the steamed artichokes with lemon immediately, with the remaining lemon wedges on the side.

The key anti•inflammatory ingredients in this recipe are:

• Artichokes: Rich in antioxidants and anti•inflammatory compounds like cynarin and silymarin.
• Lemon: Contains vitamin C and citric acid, which have anti•inflammatory properties.
• Olive oil: Provides healthy monounsaturated fats with anti•inflammatory benefits.

This simple, flavorful steamed artichoke dish is a great way to enjoy the health benefits of anti•inflammatory foods. The lemon and olive oil complement the natural sweetness of the artichokes, making this a delicious and nourishing side dish.

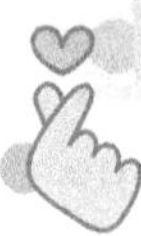

Procedure:

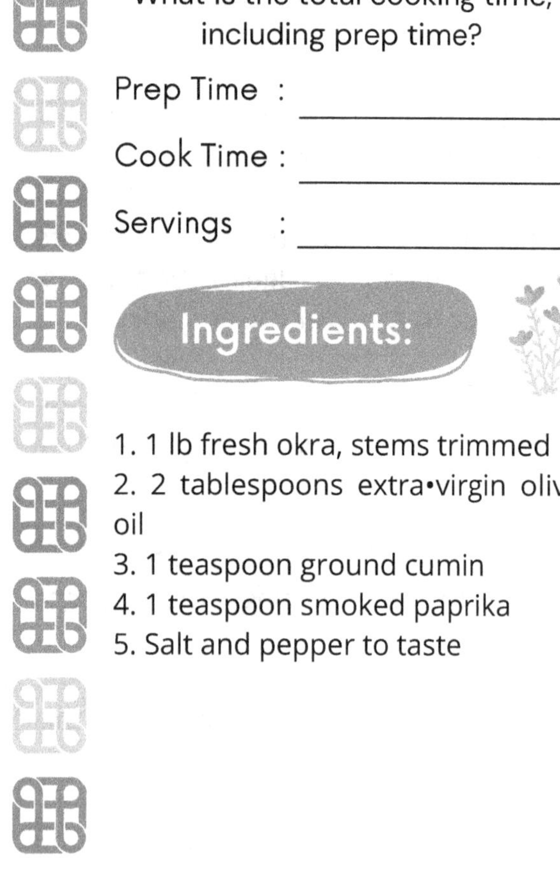

What is the total cooking time, including prep time?

Prep Time : _______________

Cook Time : _______________

Servings : _______________

Ingredients:

1. 1 lb fresh okra, stems trimmed
2. 2 tablespoons extra•virgin olive oil
3. 1 teaspoon ground cumin
4. 1 teaspoon smoked paprika
5. Salt and pepper to taste

Is the recipe easy to follow?

59. Grilled okra with cumin

1. Preheat your grill or grill pan to medium•high heat.

2. In a large bowl, toss the trimmed okra with the olive oil, cumin, smoked paprika, salt, and pepper until the okra is evenly coated.

3. Arrange the seasoned okra in a single layer on the preheated grill or grill pan.

4. Grill the okra for 5•7 minutes per side, or until it's tender and lightly charred.

5. Remove the grilled okra from the heat and transfer it to a serving platter.

6. Serve the warm, grilled okra immediately.

The key anti•inflammatory ingredients in this recipe are:

• Okra: Contains antioxidants and anti•inflammatory compounds like vitamin C, vitamin K, and polyphenols.
• Olive oil: Provides healthy monounsaturated fats with anti•inflammatory benefits.
• Cumin: Has potent anti•inflammatory and antioxidant properties.
• Smoked paprika: Contains capsaicin, which has anti•inflammatory effects.

This simple, flavorful grilled okra dish is a great way to enjoy the health benefits of anti•inflammatory foods. The smoky, spiced flavors pair perfectly with the tender, charred okra.

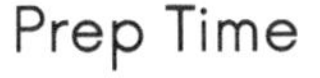

What is the total cooking time, including prep time?

Prep Time : ___________________

Cook Time : ___________________

Servings   : ___________________

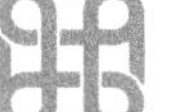

Ingredients:

1. 2 medium fennel bulbs, trimmed and cut into 1/2•inch thick slices
2. 2 tablespoons extra•virgin olive oil
3. 1 teaspoon dried thyme
4. 1 teaspoon lemon zest
5. Salt and pepper to taste

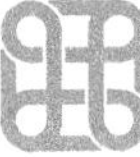

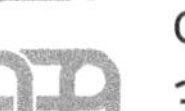

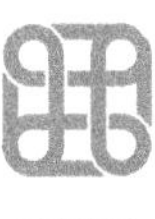

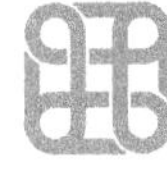

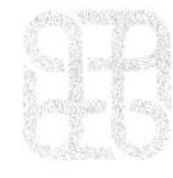

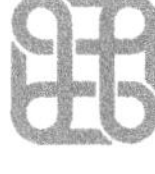

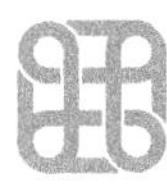

Is the recipe easy to follow?

60. Roasted fennel with olive oil

Procedure:

1. Preheat your oven to 400°F (200°C).

2. In a large bowl, toss the sliced fennel with the olive oil, dried thyme, lemon zest, salt, and pepper until the fennel is evenly coated.

3. Spread the seasoned fennel slices in a single layer on a baking sheet lined with parchment paper.

4. Roast the fennel for 20•25 minutes, flipping halfway through, until it's tender and lightly browned.

5. Remove the roasted fennel from the oven and transfer it to a serving dish.

6. Serve the warm, roasted fennel immediately.

The key anti•inflammatory ingredients in this recipe are:

• Fennel: Contains anti•inflammatory compounds like anethole and quercetin.
• Olive oil: Provides healthy monounsaturated fats with anti•inflammatory benefits.
• Thyme: Has strong anti•inflammatory and antioxidant properties.
• Lemon zest: Contains vitamin C and citric acid, which have anti•inflammatory effects.

This simple, flavorful roasted fennel dish is a great way to incorporate anti•inflammatory foods into your diet. The combination of the sweet, licorice•like fennel and the aromatic herbs and citrus makes for a delicious and nourishing side dish.

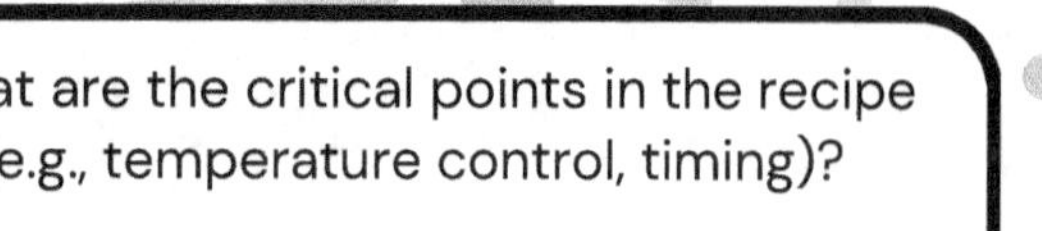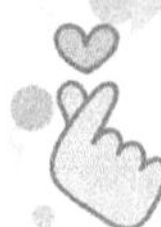

What are the critical points in the recipe (e.g., temperature control, timing)?

Procedure:

1. Preheat your oven to 400°F (200°C).

2. Line a baking sheet with parchment paper.

3. In a large bowl, toss the sliced plantains with the melted coconut oil, cinnamon, and a pinch of salt until the plantains are evenly coated.

4. Arrange the seasoned plantain slices in a single layer on the prepared baking sheet.

5. Bake for 20•25 minutes, flipping the plantains halfway through, until they are tender and lightly caramelized.

6. Remove the baked plantains from the oven and drizzle with the honey, if using.

7. Serve the warm, cinnamon•baked plantains immediately.

This simple recipe highlights the natural sweetness of ripe plantains, which are enhanced by the warmth of the cinnamon and the optional honey drizzle. The coconut oil helps to create a crispy exterior while keeping the interior soft and creamy.

Plantains are a great source of dietary fiber, vitamins, and minerals, making this a nutritious and satisfying snack or side dish. The cinnamon also provides some anti•inflammatory benefits.

You can enjoy these baked plantains on their own or use them as a topping for yogurt, oatmeal, or other dishes. They're a versatile and delicious way to incorporate more plant•based foods into your diet.

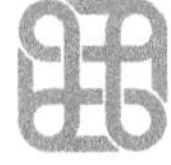

What is the total cooking time, including prep time?

Prep Time : _________________

Cook Time : _________________

Servings : _________________

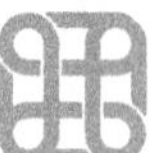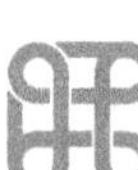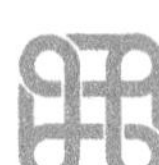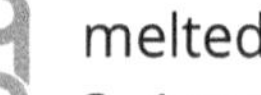

Ingredients:

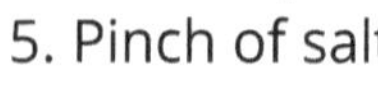

1. 2 ripe plantains, peeled and sliced diagonally into 1/2•inch thick pieces
2. 2 tablespoons coconut oil, melted
3. 1 teaspoon ground cinnamon
4. 1 tablespoon honey (optional)
5. Pinch of salt

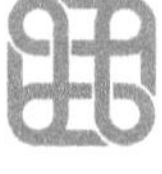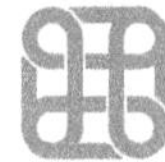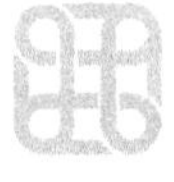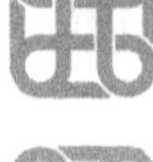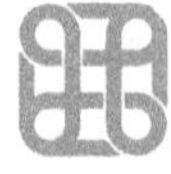

Is the recipe easy to follow?

61. Baked plantains with cinnamon

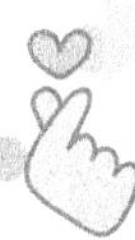

What is the total cooking time, including prep time?

Prep Time : _______________

Cook Time : _______________

Servings   : _______________

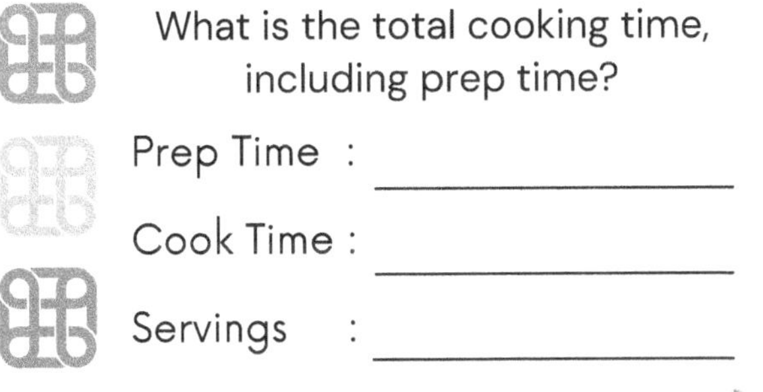

Ingredients:

1. 1 head of green cabbage, shredded or thinly sliced
2. 1 tablespoon extra•virgin olive oil
3. 1 teaspoon caraway seeds
4. 1 tablespoon apple cider vinegar
5. Salt and pepper to taste

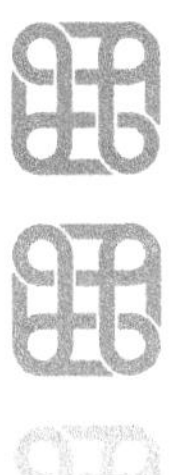
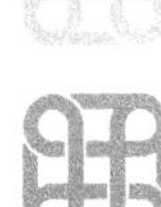
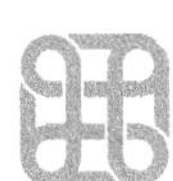

Is the recipe easy to follow?

62. Steamed cabbage with caraway seeds

1. Fill a large pot with about 1 inch of water and bring it to a boil over high heat.

2. Add the shredded or sliced cabbage to a steamer basket and place it in the pot. Cover and steam the cabbage for 5•7 minutes, or until it's tender but still crisp.

3. Drain the steamed cabbage and transfer it to a serving bowl.

4. Drizzle the olive oil over the hot cabbage and sprinkle the caraway seeds on top. Toss to coat the cabbage evenly.

5. Drizzle the apple cider vinegar over the cabbage and season with salt and pepper to taste.

6. Serve the steamed cabbage with caraway seeds warm.

The key anti•inflammatory ingredients in this recipe are:

• Cabbage: A cruciferous vegetable rich in antioxidants and anti•inflammatory compounds like sulforaphane and vitamin C.
• Olive oil: Provides healthy monounsaturated fats with anti•inflammatory benefits.
• Caraway seeds: Contain anti•inflammatory compounds like carvone and limonene.
• Apple cider vinegar: Has anti•inflammatory properties due to its acetic acid content.

This simple, flavorful steamed cabbage dish is a great way to incorporate anti•inflammatory foods into your diet. Enjoy it as a side dish or add it to soups, stews, or other meals.

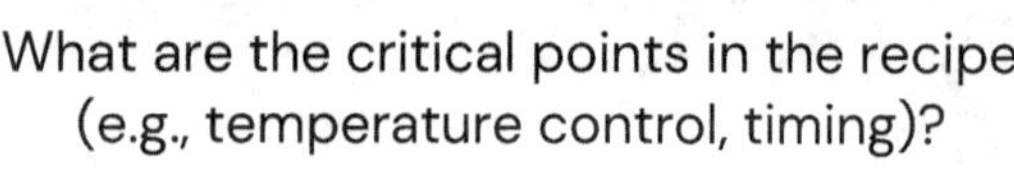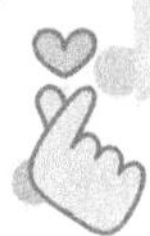

What are the critical points in the recipe (e.g., temperature control, timing)?

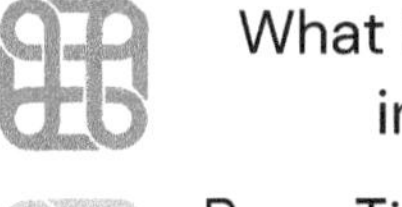

What is the total cooking time, including prep time?

Prep Time : ___________________

Cook Time : ___________________

Servings   : ___________________

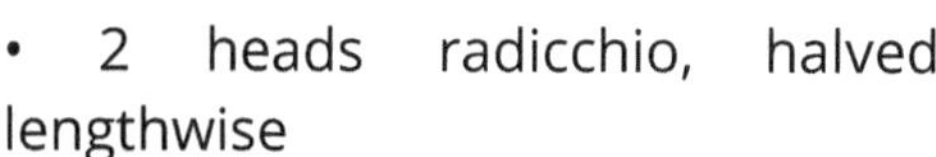

- 2 heads radicchio, halved lengthwise
- 2 tbsp olive oil
- 2 tbsp balsamic vinegar
- Salt and pepper to taste

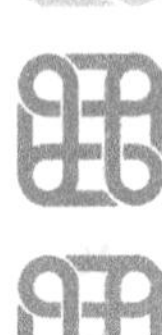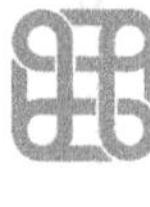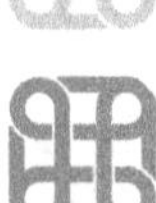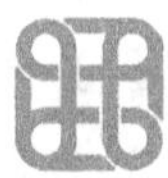

Is the recipe easy to follow?

63. *Grilled radicchio with balsamic*

1. Preheat grill or grill pan to medium•high heat.

2. Brush the cut sides of the radicchio halves with olive oil. Season with salt and pepper.

3. Place the radicchio halves cut•side down on the grill. Grill for 2•3 minutes per side, until charred and slightly softened.

4. Transfer the grilled radicchio to a serving platter. Drizzle with balsamic vinegar.

5. Serve immediately, while the radicchio is still warm. The balsamic vinegar will create a nice glaze on the grilled radicchio.

The bitterness of the radicchio pairs beautifully with the sweet and tangy balsamic vinegar. This makes a great side dish or appetizer. Enjoy!

What are the critical points in the recipe (e.g., temperature control, timing)?

What is the total cooking time, including prep time?

Prep Time : ___________________

Cook Time : ___________________

Servings   : ___________________

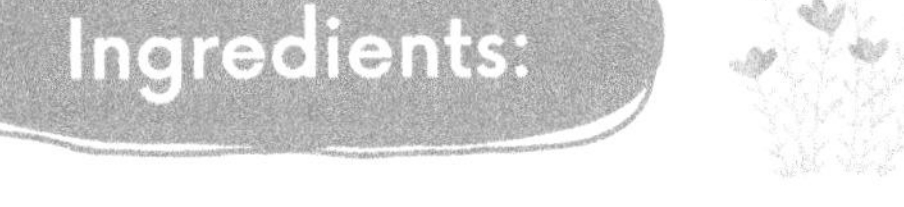

Ingredients:

• 4 large portobello mushroom caps, stems removed
• 2 tbsp extra•virgin olive oil
• 2 tsp dried oregano
• 1 tsp dried thyme
• 1/2 tsp sea salt

Is the recipe easy to follow?

64. Baked portobello caps with herbs

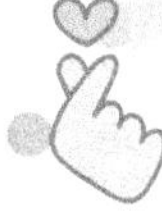

Procedure:

1. Preheat oven to 400°F (200°C).

2. Gently wipe the portobello caps clean with a damp paper towel. Remove the stems and discard.

3. In a small bowl, combine the olive oil, oregano, thyme, and sea salt. Stir to mix well.

4. Arrange the portobello caps gill•side up on a baking sheet. Brush the tops generously with the herb•oil mixture, making sure to coat the caps completely.

5. Bake for 12•15 minutes, until the mushrooms are tender and lightly browned.

6. Serve the baked portobello caps warm, as a side dish or appetizer.

The key anti•inflammatory ingredients in this recipe are:

• Portobello mushrooms • contain antioxidants and anti•inflammatory compounds
• Olive oil • a healthy fat with anti•inflammatory properties
• Oregano and thyme • herbs with potent anti•inflammatory effects

This simple 5•ingredient dish makes a great option for an easy, healthy, and anti•inflammatory meal or snack. Enjoy!

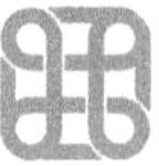 What is the total cooking time,
including prep time?

Prep Time : _______________

Cook Time : _______________

Servings   : _______________

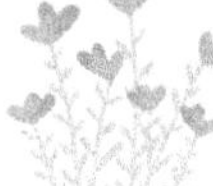

Ingredients:

1. 1 lb turnips, peeled and cut into
1•inch cubes
2. 2 tbsp olive oil
3. 1 tsp dried thyme
4. 1/2 tsp salt
5. 1/4 tsp black pepper

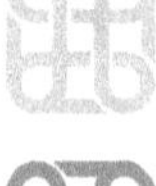
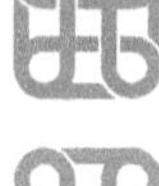
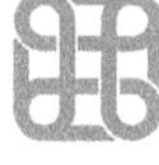
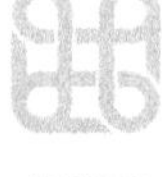
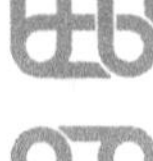
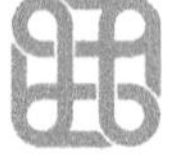

**Is the recipe easy to
follow?**

65. Roasted turnips with thyme

Procedure:

2. In a large bowl, toss the cubed turnips with the olive oil, thyme, salt, and pepper until evenly coated.
3. Spread the turnips in a single layer on a baking sheet.
4. Roast for 25•30 minutes, flipping halfway, until the turnips are tender and lightly browned.
5. Serve hot.

The key anti•inflammatory ingredients in this recipe are:

1. Turnips • Contain antioxidants and anti•inflammatory compounds like vitamin C.

2. Olive oil • Rich in monounsaturated fats that have anti•inflammatory properties.

3. Thyme • Contains the compound thymol, which has potent anti•inflammatory effects.

This simple 5•ingredient side dish is a great way to incorporate more anti•inflammatory foods into your diet.

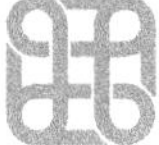

What is the total cooking time, including prep time?

Prep Time : _________________

Cook Time : _________________

Servings : _________________

Ingredients:

• 4 heads of endive, halved lengthwise
• 2 tbsp extra•virgin olive oil
• 1 tsp lemon juice
• 1/2 tsp sea salt
• 1/4 tsp ground black pepper

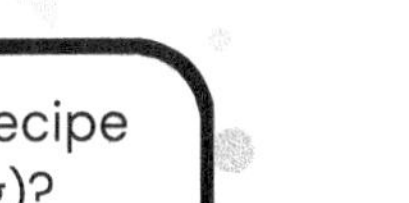

Procedure:

1. Preheat grill or grill pan to medium•high heat.

2. In a small bowl, whisk together the olive oil, lemon juice, salt, and pepper.

3. Brush the cut sides of the endive halves with the olive oil mixture, making sure to coat them evenly.

4. Place the endive halves, cut•side down, on the preheated grill. Grill for 2•3 minutes per side, until lightly charred and tender.

5. Transfer the grilled endive to a serving platter. Drizzle any remaining olive oil mixture over the top.

6. Serve the grilled endive warm or at room temperature.

The key anti•inflammatory ingredients in this recipe are:

• Endive • contains antioxidants and anti•inflammatory compounds
• Olive oil • a healthy fat with potent anti•inflammatory properties
• Lemon juice • provides vitamin C and has anti•inflammatory effects

This simple 5•ingredient grilled endive dish makes a great side or appetizer option for an easy, healthy, and anti•inflammatory meal. Enjoy!

Is the recipe easy to follow?

66. Grilled endive with olive oil

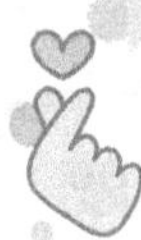

Procedure:

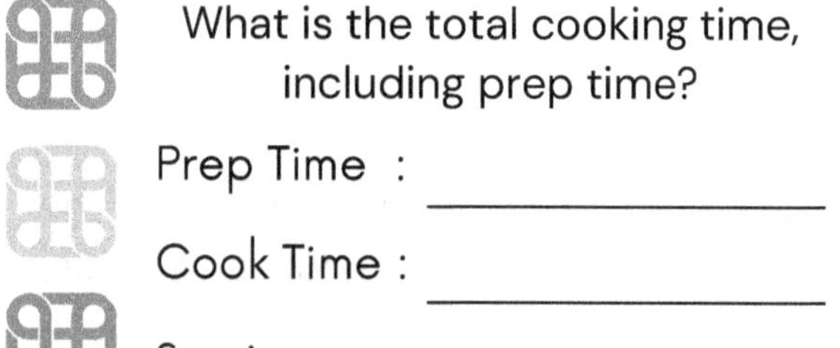

What is the total cooking time, including prep time?

Prep Time : _______________

Cook Time : _______________

Servings   : _______________

Ingredients:

• 2 lbs rutabaga, peeled and cut into 1/2•inch thick fry shapes
• 2 tbsp extra•virgin olive oil
• 1 tsp ground turmeric
• 1 tsp ground cumin
• 1/2 tsp sea salt

1. Preheat oven to 400°F (200°C). Line a large baking sheet with parchment paper.

2. In a large bowl, toss the rutabaga fries with the olive oil, turmeric, cumin, and sea salt until evenly coated.

3. Spread the seasoned rutabaga fries in a single layer on the prepared baking sheet.

4. Bake for 25•30 minutes, flipping halfway, until the fries are tender and lightly browned.

5. Remove the baked rutabaga fries from the oven and serve hot.

The key anti•inflammatory ingredients in this recipe are:

• Rutabaga • a root vegetable rich in antioxidants and anti•inflammatory compounds
• Olive oil • a healthy fat with potent anti•inflammatory properties
• Turmeric • a spice with powerful anti•inflammatory effects
• Cumin • a spice with anti•inflammatory and antioxidant benefits

This simple 5•ingredient baked rutabaga fries dish makes a great side or snack option for an easy, healthy, and anti•inflammatory meal. Enjoy!

Is the recipe easy to follow?

67. Baked rutabaga fries

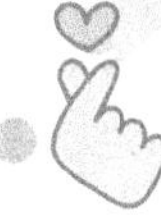

What are the critical points in the recipe (e.g., temperature control, timing)?

What is the total cooking time, including prep time?

Prep Time : _________________

Cook Time : _________________

Servings : _________________

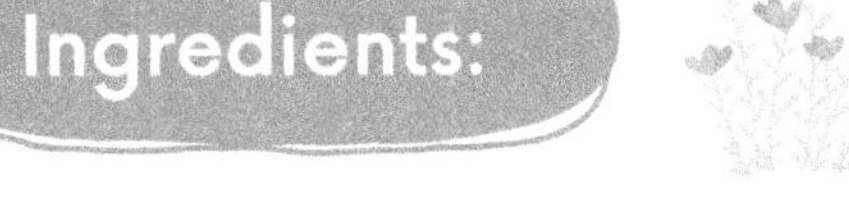

Ingredients:

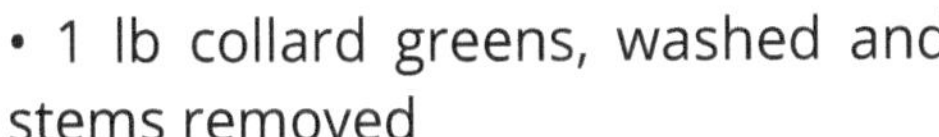

• 1 lb collard greens, washed and stems removed
• 2 tbsp extra•virgin olive oil
• 3 cloves garlic, minced
• 1 tsp apple cider vinegar
• 1/4 tsp sea salt

1. Fill a large pot with 1•2 inches of water and bring to a boil over high heat.

2. Add the collard green leaves to a steamer basket and place the basket in the pot. Cover and steam for 5•7 minutes, until the greens are tender.

3. In a small bowl, whisk together the olive oil, minced garlic, apple cider vinegar, and sea salt.

4. Transfer the steamed collard greens to a serving bowl. Drizzle the garlic•vinegar dressing over the top and toss to coat.

5. Serve the steamed collard greens warm.

The key anti•inflammatory ingredients in this recipe are:

• Collard greens • a leafy green packed with antioxidants and anti•inflammatory compounds
• Olive oil • a healthy fat with potent anti•inflammatory properties
• Garlic • a potent anti•inflammatory food
• Apple cider vinegar • contains acetic acid with anti•inflammatory benefits

This simple 5•ingredient steamed collard greens dish makes a great side or addition to any anti•inflammatory meal. Enjoy!

Is the recipe easy to follow?

68. Steamed collard greens with garlic

What are the critical points in the recipe (e.g., temperature control, timing)?

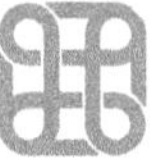 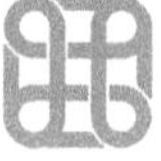

What is the total cooking time, including prep time?

Prep Time : ______________

Cook Time : ______________

Servings   : ______________

 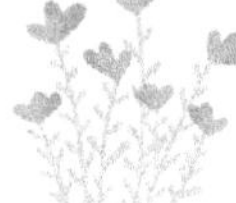

Ingredients:

• 4 heads of Belgian endive, halved lengthwise
• 2 tablespoons olive oil
• 1 tablespoon balsamic vinegar
• Salt and pepper to taste

Is the recipe easy to follow?

69. Grilled Belgian endive

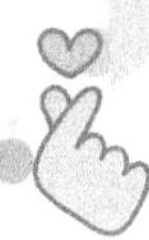

Procedure:

1. Preheat your grill or grill pan to medium•high heat.

2. Brush the cut sides of the endive halves with the olive oil, making sure to coat them evenly.

3. Season the endive halves with salt and pepper.

4. Place the endive halves, cut•side down, on the preheated grill. Grill for 2•3 minutes per side, until lightly charred and tender.

5. Transfer the grilled endive to a serving platter. Drizzle the balsamic vinegar over the top.

6. Serve the grilled Belgian endive warm or at room temperature.

The grilling process caramelizes the natural sugars in the endive, creating a delicious sweet and slightly bitter flavor. The balsamic vinegar adds a nice tangy note to balance out the flavors.

This simple grilled endive dish makes a great side or appetizer. It pairs well with grilled meats, fish, or as part of a larger salad or vegetable platter.

Enjoy the smoky, caramelized goodness of the grilled Belgian endive!

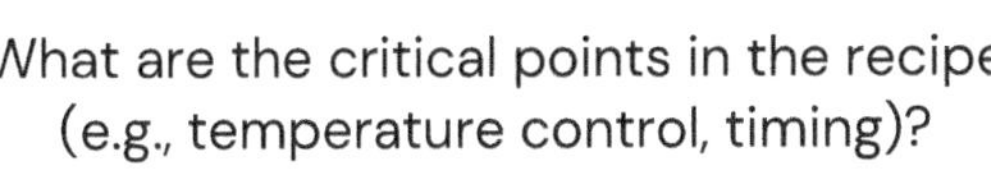

What are the critical points in the recipe (e.g., temperature control, timing)?

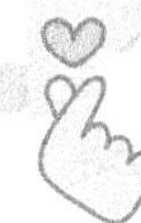

What is the total cooking time, including prep time?

Prep Time : _________________

Cook Time : _________________

Servings   : _________________

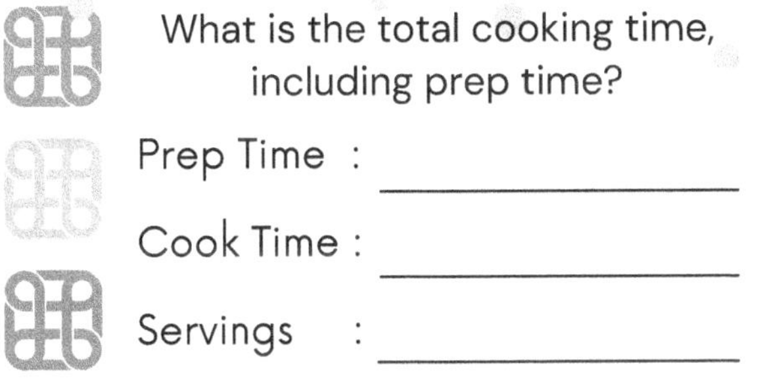

1. 2 medium kohlrabi bulbs, peeled and cut into 1•inch cubes
2. 2 tablespoons extra•virgin olive oil
3. 1 teaspoon dried thyme
4. 1 teaspoon lemon zest
5. Salt and pepper to taste

Is the recipe easy to follow?

70. Roasted kohlrabi with olive oil

1. Preheat your oven to 400°F (200°C).

2. In a large bowl, toss the cubed kohlrabi with the olive oil, dried thyme, lemon zest, salt, and pepper until the kohlrabi is evenly coated.

3. Spread the seasoned kohlrabi cubes in a single layer on a baking sheet lined with parchment paper.

4. Roast the kohlrabi for 20•25 minutes, flipping halfway through, until it's tender and lightly browned.

5. Remove the roasted kohlrabi from the oven and transfer it to a serving dish.

6. Serve the warm, roasted kohlrabi immediately.

The key anti•inflammatory ingredients in this recipe are:

• Kohlrabi: A cruciferous vegetable that contains anti•inflammatory compounds like glucosinolates and vitamin C.
• Olive oil: Provides healthy monounsaturated fats with anti•inflammatory benefits.
• Thyme: Has strong anti•inflammatory and antioxidant properties.
• Lemon zest: Contains vitamin C and citric acid, which have anti•inflammatory effects.

This simple, flavorful roasted kohlrabi dish is a great way to incorporate anti•inflammatory foods into your diet. The combination of the earthy kohlrabi, aromatic herbs, and bright citrus makes for a delicious and nourishing side dish.

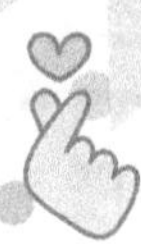

What are the critical points in the recipe (e.g., temperature control, timing)?

 What is the total cooking time, including prep time?

Prep Time : ___________________

Cook Time : ___________________

Servings : ___________________

Ingredients:

• 1 lb parsnips, peeled and sliced into 1/8•inch thick rounds
• 2 tbsp olive oil
• 1 tsp salt
• 1/2 tsp black pepper

Is the recipe easy to follow?

71. Baked parsnip chips

Procedure:

1. Preheat your oven to 400°F (200°C). Line two baking sheets with parchment paper.

2. In a large bowl, toss the parsnip slices with the olive oil, salt, and black pepper until evenly coated.

3. Arrange the seasoned parsnip slices in a single layer on the prepared baking sheets, making sure they are not overlapping.

4. Bake for 20•25 minutes, flipping the parsnip chips halfway, until they are golden brown and crispy.

5. Remove the baked parsnip chips from the oven and let cool for a few minutes.

6. Serve the parsnip chips warm or at room temperature.

Tips:
• Make sure to slice the parsnips evenly to ensure even cooking.
• Adjust the baking time as needed, keeping a close eye on the chips to prevent burning.
• For extra crispiness, you can bake the chips in batches.

Parsnips are a root vegetable that are naturally sweet and starchy, making them the perfect base for homemade baked chips. The combination of olive oil, salt, and pepper creates a delicious, savory flavor.

These baked parsnip chips make a great healthy snack or side dish. Enjoy their crispy texture and natural sweetness!

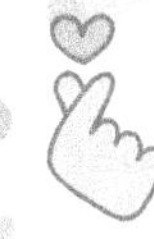

Procedure:

Prep Time : _______________

Cook Time : _______________

Servings   : _______________

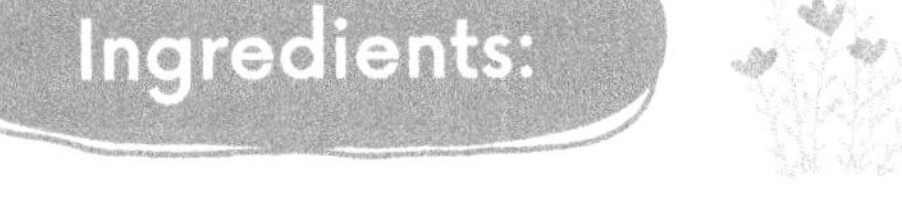

Ingredients:

• 1 lb mustard greens, washed and stems removed
• 1 tbsp sesame oil
• 2 tsp grated fresh ginger
• 1 tbsp low•sodium soy sauce or tamari
• 1 tsp rice vinegar
• Salt and pepper to taste

1. Fill a large pot with 1•2 inches of water and bring to a boil over high heat.

2. Add the mustard greens to a steamer basket and place the basket in the pot. Cover and steam for 5•7 minutes, until the greens are tender.

3. In a small bowl, whisk together the sesame oil, grated ginger, soy sauce, and rice vinegar.

4. Transfer the steamed mustard greens to a serving bowl. Drizzle the ginger•soy dressing over the top and toss to coat.

5. Season with salt and pepper to taste.

6. Serve the steamed mustard greens warm.

The ginger and soy sauce provide a nice balance of heat and umami flavors that complement the slightly bitter and peppery taste of the mustard greens. The steaming process helps to tenderize the greens and preserve their nutrients.

This simple dish makes a great side or addition to any Asian•inspired meal. The mustard greens are packed with vitamins, minerals, and antioxidants, making it a nutritious and anti•inflammatory option.

Enjoy the bright, flavorful combination of the steamed mustard greens and ginger!

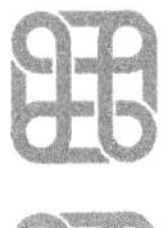
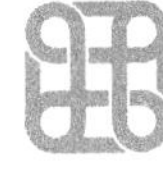
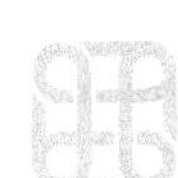
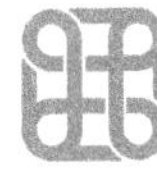
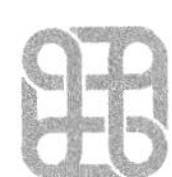

Is the recipe easy to follow?

72. *Steamed mustard greens with ginger*

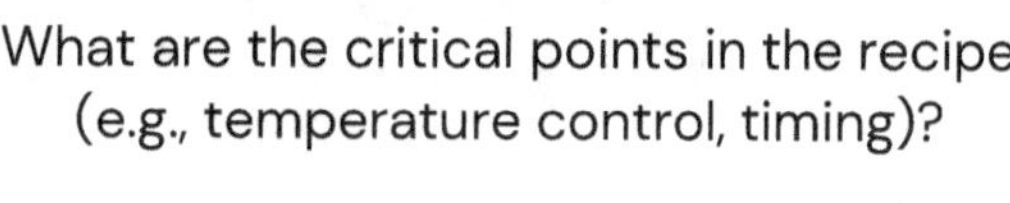

What are the critical points in the recipe (e.g., temperature control, timing)?

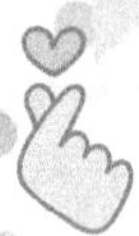

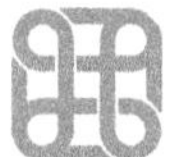

What is the total cooking time, including prep time?

Prep Time : _______________

Cook Time : _______________

Servings   : _______________

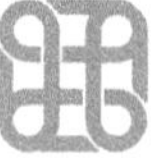 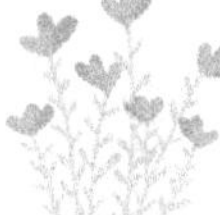

Ingredients:

• 4 large leeks, white and light green parts only, halved lengthwise
• 2 tablespoons extra•virgin olive oil
• 1 tablespoon fresh lemon juice
• 1/2 teaspoon sea salt
• 1/4 teaspoon ground black pepper

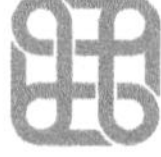
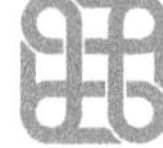
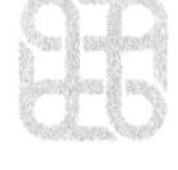
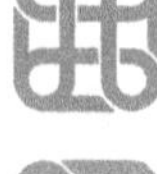
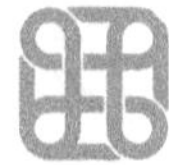

Is the recipe easy to follow?

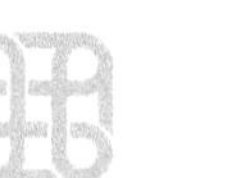  

73. Grilled leeks with lemon

1. Preheat your grill or grill pan to medium•high heat.

2. In a small bowl, whisk together the olive oil, lemon juice, salt, and pepper.

3. Brush the cut sides of the leek halves with the lemon•oil mixture, making sure to coat them evenly.

4. Place the leek halves, cut•side down, on the preheated grill. Grill for 3•5 minutes per side, until lightly charred and tender.

5. Transfer the grilled leeks to a serving platter. Drizzle any remaining lemon•oil mixture over the top.

6. Serve the grilled leeks warm or at room temperature.

The key anti•inflammatory ingredients in this recipe are:

• Leeks • contain antioxidants and anti•inflammatory compounds
• Olive oil • a healthy fat with potent anti•inflammatory properties
• Lemon juice • provides vitamin C and has anti•inflammatory effects

This simple 5•ingredient grilled leeks dish makes a great side or appetizer option for an easy, healthy, and anti•inflammatory meal. Enjoy!

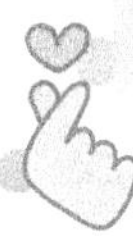

What are the critical points in the recipe (e.g., temperature control, timing)?

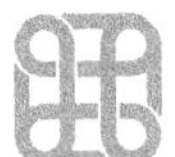

What is the total cooking time, including prep time?

Prep Time : _______________

Cook Time : _______________

Servings   : _______________

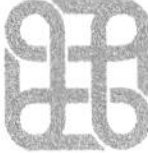

Ingredients:

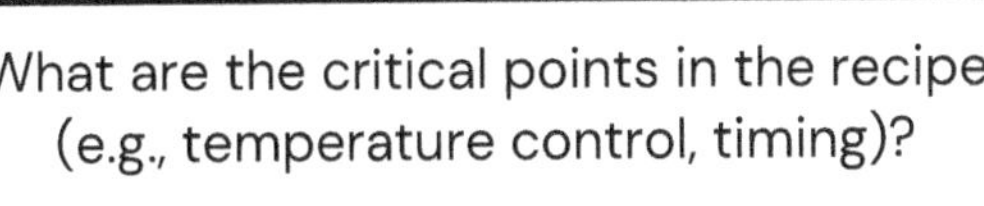

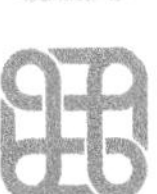

• 1 medium spaghetti squash, halved lengthwise and seeds removed
• 2 tbsp extra•virgin olive oil
• 1 tsp dried oregano
• 1 tsp dried basil
• 1/2 tsp sea salt

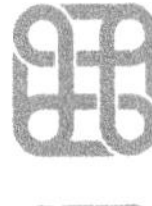

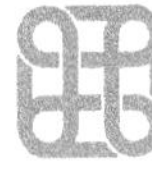

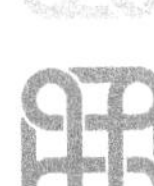

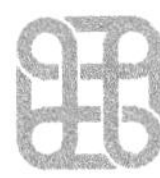

Is the recipe easy to follow?

74. Baked spaghetti squash with herbs

1. Preheat your oven to 400°F (200°C). Line a baking sheet with parchment paper.

2. Place the spaghetti squash halves cut•side up on the prepared baking sheet.

3. In a small bowl, combine the olive oil, oregano, basil, and sea salt. Stir to mix well.

4. Brush the cut sides of the spaghetti squash halves with the herb•oil mixture, making sure to coat them evenly.

5. Bake for 40•50 minutes, until the squash is tender and easily shreds with a fork.

6. Remove the baked spaghetti squash from the oven and let cool slightly. Use a fork to shred the flesh into strands.

7. Transfer the spaghetti squash strands to a serving bowl. Drizzle any remaining herb•oil mixture over the top.

8. Serve the baked spaghetti squash warm.

The key anti•inflammatory ingredients in this recipe are:

• Spaghetti squash • a winter squash rich in antioxidants and anti•inflammatory compounds
• Olive oil • a healthy fat with potent anti•inflammatory properties
• Oregano and basil • herbs with powerful anti•inflammatory effects

This simple 5•ingredient baked spaghetti squash dish makes a great side or base for an easy, healthy, and anti•inflammatory meal. Enjoy!

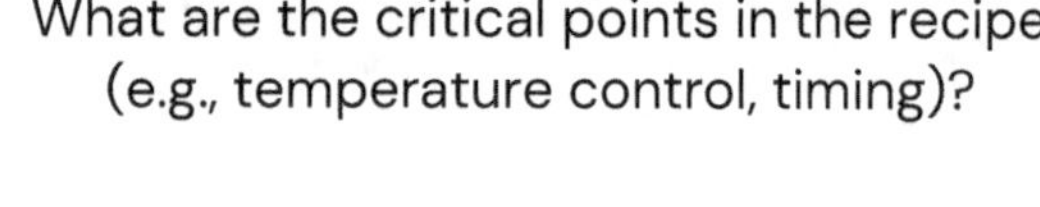
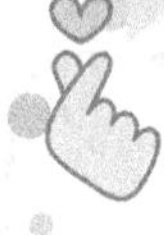

What are the critical points in the recipe (e.g., temperature control, timing)?

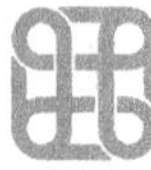

What is the total cooking time, including prep time?

Prep Time : ________________

Cook Time : ________________

Servings   : ________________

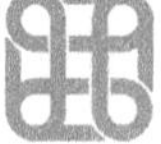

Ingredients:

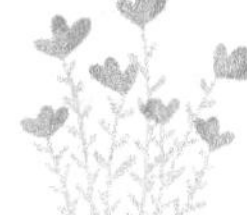

• 2 lbs celery root, peeled and cut into 1•inch cubes
• 2 tbsp extra•virgin olive oil
• 1 tsp dried thyme
• 1/2 tsp sea salt
• 1/4 tsp ground black pepper

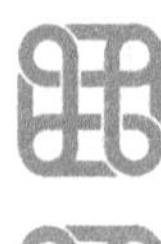
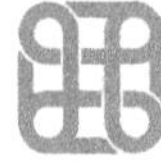
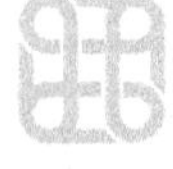
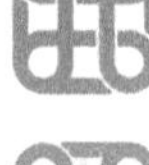

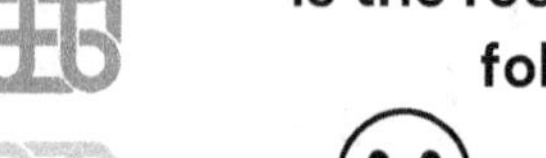

Is the recipe easy to follow?

75. Roasted celery root with thyme

Procedure:

1. Preheat your oven to 400°F (200°C). Line a large baking sheet with parchment paper.

2. In a large bowl, toss the celery root cubes with the olive oil, dried thyme, sea salt, and black pepper until evenly coated.

3. Spread the seasoned celery root in a single layer on the prepared baking sheet.

4. Roast for 25•30 minutes, flipping the celery root halfway, until tender and lightly browned.

5. Remove the roasted celery root from the oven and serve warm.

The key anti•inflammatory ingredients in this recipe are:

• Celery root • a root vegetable rich in antioxidants and anti•inflammatory compounds
• Olive oil • a healthy fat with potent anti•inflammatory properties
• Thyme • an herb with powerful anti•inflammatory effects

This simple 5•ingredient roasted celery root dish makes a great side or addition to any anti•inflammatory meal. Enjoy!

What are the critical points in the recipe (e.g., temperature control, timing)?

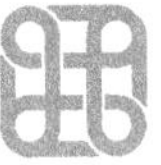 **What is the total cooking time, including prep time?**

Prep Time : _______________

Cook Time : _______________

Servings   : _______________

 **Ingredients:**

• 1 lb rapini (also called broccoli rabe), tough stems removed
• 2 tbsp extra•virgin olive oil
• 3 cloves garlic, minced
• 1 tbsp lemon juice
• 1/4 tsp sea salt

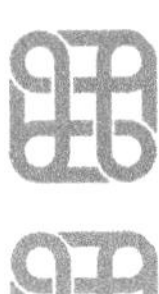
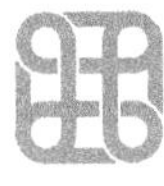
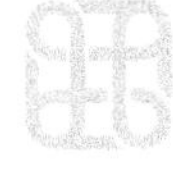
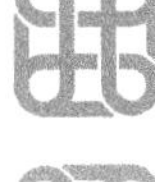
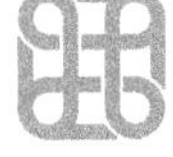

Is the recipe easy to follow?

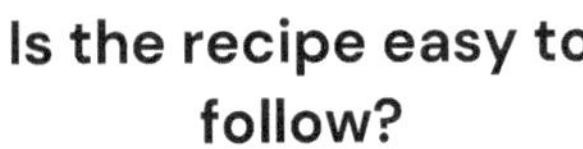

76. *Grilled rapini with garlic*

1. Preheat your grill or grill pan to medium•high heat.

2. In a large bowl, toss the rapini with the olive oil, minced garlic, lemon juice, and sea salt until evenly coated.

3. Arrange the seasoned rapini in a single layer on the preheated grill. Grill for 2•3 minutes per side, until lightly charred and tender.

4. Transfer the grilled rapini to a serving platter.

5. Serve the grilled rapini warm, garnished with any remaining garlic•lemon oil from the bowl.

The key anti•inflammatory ingredients in this recipe are:

• Rapini • a cruciferous vegetable rich in antioxidants and anti•inflammatory compounds
• Olive oil • a healthy fat with potent anti•inflammatory properties
• Garlic • a potent anti•inflammatory food
• Lemon juice • provides vitamin C and has anti•inflammatory effects

This simple 5•ingredient grilled rapini dish makes a great side or addition to any anti•inflammatory meal. Enjoy!

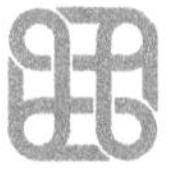

What is the total cooking time, including prep time?

Prep Time : ______________

Cook Time : ______________

Servings : ______________

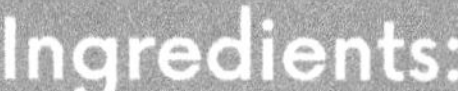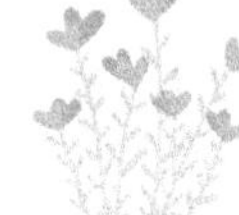

Ingredients:

• 2 lbs jicama, peeled and cut into 1/2•inch thick fry shapes
• 2 tbsp extra•virgin olive oil
• 1 tsp ground cumin
• 1 tsp smoked paprika
• 1/2 tsp sea salt

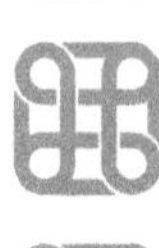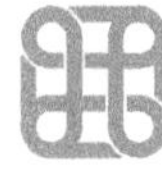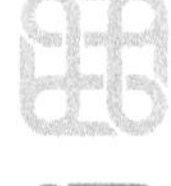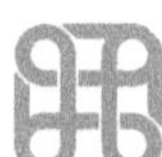

Is the recipe easy to follow?

77. Baked jicama fries

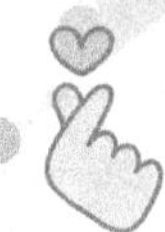

Procedure:

1. Preheat oven to 400°F (200°C). Line a large baking sheet with parchment paper.

2. In a large bowl, toss the jicama fries with the olive oil, cumin, smoked paprika, and sea salt until evenly coated.

3. Spread the seasoned jicama fries in a single layer on the prepared baking sheet.

4. Bake for 25•30 minutes, flipping halfway, until the fries are tender and lightly browned.

5. Remove the baked jicama fries from the oven and serve hot.

The key anti•inflammatory ingredients in this recipe are:

• Jicama • a root vegetable rich in antioxidants and anti•inflammatory compounds
• Olive oil • a healthy fat with potent anti•inflammatory properties
• Cumin • a spice with anti•inflammatory and antioxidant benefits
• Smoked paprika • a spice with anti•inflammatory effects

This simple 5•ingredient baked jicama fries dish makes a great side or snack option for an easy, healthy, and anti•inflammatory meal. Enjoy!

What is the total cooking time, including prep time?

Prep Time : _______________

Cook Time : _______________

Servings   : _______________

Ingredients:

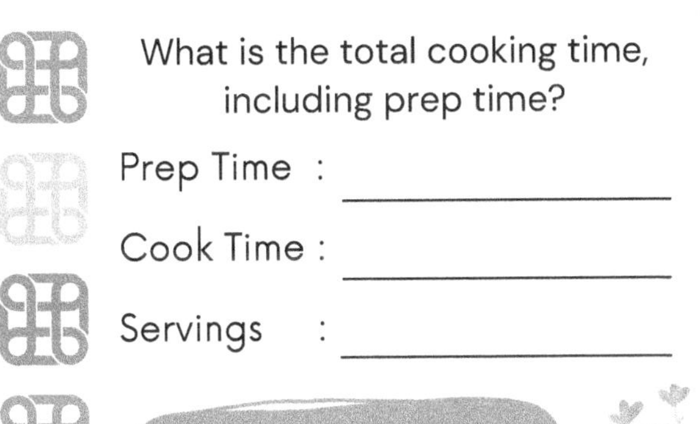

• 1 lb dandelion greens, washed and stems removed
• 2 tbsp extra•virgin olive oil
• 2 tbsp fresh lemon juice
• 1 tsp Dijon mustard
• 1/4 tsp sea salt

Is the recipe easy to follow?

78. Steamed dandelion greens with lemon

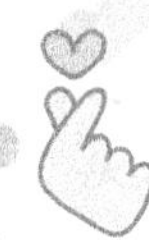

Procedure:

1. Fill a large pot with 1•2 inches of water and bring to a boil over high heat.

2. Add the dandelion greens to a steamer basket and place the basket in the pot. Cover and steam for 5•7 minutes, until the greens are tender.

3. In a small bowl, whisk together the olive oil, lemon juice, Dijon mustard, and sea salt.

4. Transfer the steamed dandelion greens to a serving bowl. Drizzle the lemon•mustard dressing over the top and toss to coat.

5. Serve the steamed dandelion greens warm.

The key anti•inflammatory ingredients in this recipe are:

• Dandelion greens • a leafy green packed with antioxidants and anti•inflammatory compounds
• Olive oil • a healthy fat with potent anti•inflammatory properties
• Lemon juice • provides vitamin C and has anti•inflammatory effects
• Dijon mustard • contains compounds with anti•inflammatory benefits

This simple 5•ingredient steamed dandelion greens dish makes a great side or addition to any anti•inflammatory meal. Enjoy!

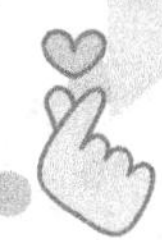

Procedure:

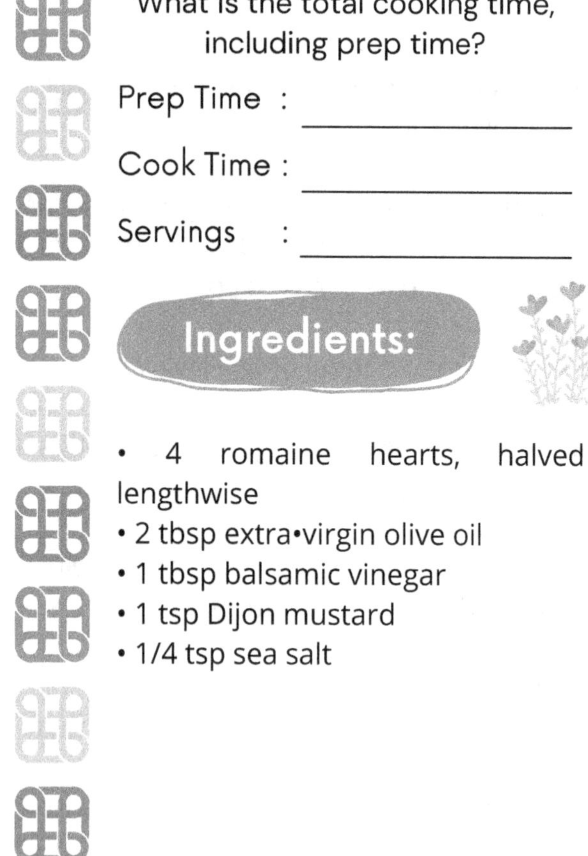

What is the total cooking time, including prep time?

Prep Time   : _________________

Cook Time : _________________

Servings   : _________________

Ingredients:

- 4 romaine hearts, halved lengthwise
- 2 tbsp extra•virgin olive oil
- 1 tbsp balsamic vinegar
- 1 tsp Dijon mustard
- 1/4 tsp sea salt

Is the recipe easy to follow?

79. Grilled romaine hearts

1. Preheat your grill or grill pan to medium•high heat.

2. In a small bowl, whisk together the olive oil, balsamic vinegar, Dijon mustard, and sea salt.

3. Brush the cut sides of the romaine hearts with the dressing mixture, making sure to coat them evenly.

4. Place the romaine hearts, cut•side down, on the preheated grill. Grill for 2•3 minutes per side, until lightly charred and slightly wilted.

5. Transfer the grilled romaine hearts to a serving platter. Drizzle any remaining dressing over the top.

6. Serve the grilled romaine hearts warm.

The key anti•inflammatory ingredients in this recipe are:

- Romaine lettuce • a leafy green with anti•inflammatory properties
- Olive oil • a healthy fat with potent anti•inflammatory effects
- Balsamic vinegar • contains compounds with anti•inflammatory benefits
- Dijon mustard • provides anti•inflammatory compounds

This simple 5•ingredient grilled romaine hearts dish makes a great side or addition to any anti•inflammatory meal. Enjoy!

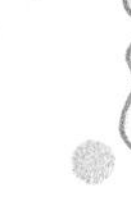

1. Preheat your oven to 400°F (200°C). Line a baking sheet with parchment paper.

2. In a large bowl, toss the Jerusalem artichoke pieces with the olive oil, dried rosemary, dried thyme, and sea salt until evenly coated.

3. Spread the seasoned Jerusalem artichokes in a single layer on the prepared baking sheet.

4. Roast for 25•30 minutes, flipping the artichokes halfway, until they are tender and lightly browned.

5. Remove the roasted Jerusalem artichokes from the oven and serve warm.

The key anti•inflammatory ingredients in this recipe are:

• Jerusalem artichokes • a root vegetable rich in antioxidants and anti•inflammatory compounds
• Olive oil • a healthy fat with potent anti•inflammatory properties
• Rosemary and thyme • herbs with powerful anti•inflammatory effects

This simple 5•ingredient roasted Jerusalem artichokes dish makes a great side or addition to any anti•inflammatory meal. Enjoy!

What is the total cooking time, including prep time?

Prep Time : _________________

Cook Time : _________________

Servings   : _________________

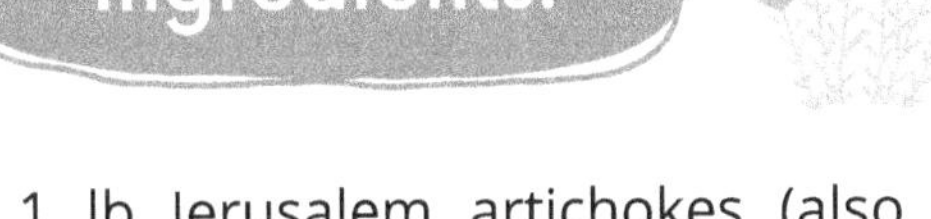
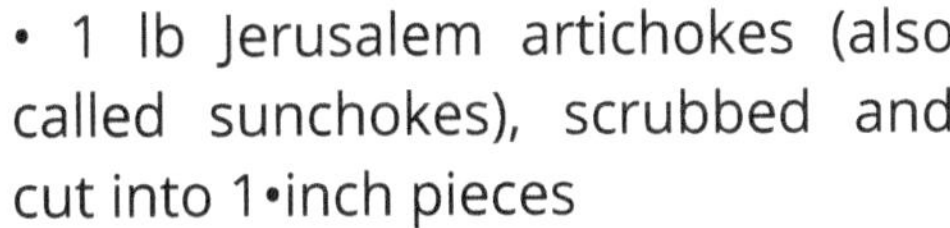

• 1 lb Jerusalem artichokes (also called sunchokes), scrubbed and cut into 1•inch pieces
• 2 tbsp extra•virgin olive oil
• 1 tsp dried rosemary
• 1 tsp dried thyme
• 1/2 tsp sea salt

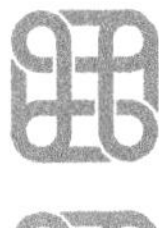
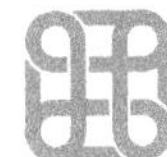
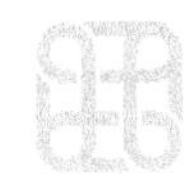
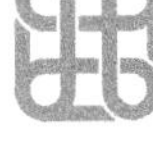
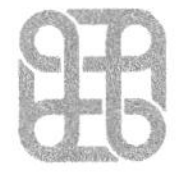

Is the recipe easy to follow?

80. Roasted Jerusalem artichokes

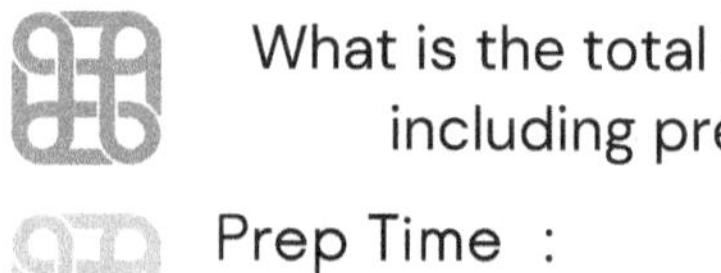

What is the total cooking time, including prep time?

Prep Time : _______________

Cook Time : _______________

Servings   : _______________

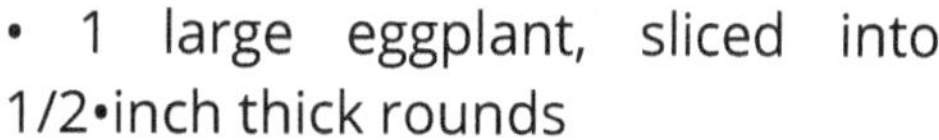

Ingredients:

• 1 large eggplant, sliced into 1/2•inch thick rounds
• 2 tablespoons extra•virgin olive oil
• 1 teaspoon dried oregano
• 1 teaspoon dried basil
• 1/2 teaspoon sea salt

Is the recipe easy to follow?

81. Baked eggplant slices with herbs

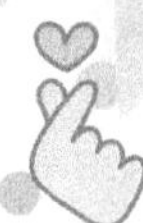

Procedure:

1. Preheat your oven to 400°F (200°C). Line a baking sheet with parchment paper.

2. In a small bowl, combine the olive oil, oregano, basil, and sea salt. Stir to mix well.

3. Arrange the eggplant slices in a single layer on the prepared baking sheet. Brush the tops of the eggplant slices with the herb•oil mixture, making sure to coat them evenly.

4. Bake for 20•25 minutes, flipping the eggplant slices halfway, until they are tender and lightly browned.

5. Remove the baked eggplant slices from the oven and serve warm.

The key anti•inflammatory ingredients in this recipe are:

• Eggplant • contains antioxidants and anti•inflammatory compounds
• Olive oil • a healthy fat with potent anti•inflammatory properties
• Oregano and basil • herbs with powerful anti•inflammatory effects

This simple 5•ingredient baked eggplant slices dish makes a great side or appetizer option for an easy, healthy, and anti•inflammatory meal. Enjoy!

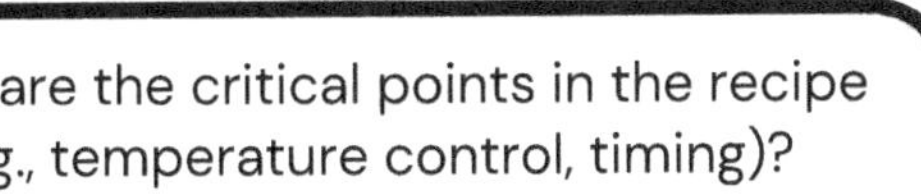

What are the critical points in the recipe (e.g., temperature control, timing)?

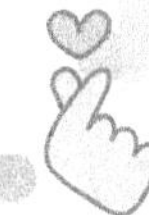

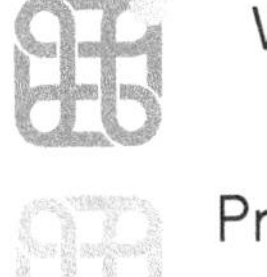

What is the total cooking time, including prep time?

Prep Time : _________________

Cook Time : _________________

Servings   : _________________

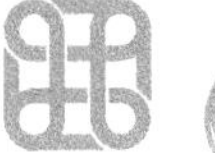

Ingredients:

• 1 lb Swiss chard, washed and stems removed
• 2 tbsp extra•virgin olive oil
• 3 cloves garlic, minced
• 1 tbsp lemon juice
• 1/4 tsp sea salt

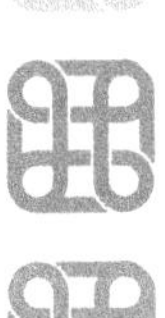

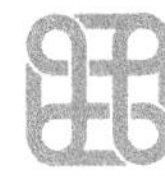

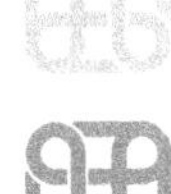

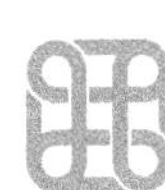

Is the recipe easy to follow?

82. Steamed chard with garlic

1. Fill a large pot with 1•2 inches of water and bring to a boil over high heat.

2. Add the chard leaves to a steamer basket and place the basket in the pot. Cover and steam for 5•7 minutes, until the chard is tender.

3. In a small bowl, whisk together the olive oil, minced garlic, lemon juice, and sea salt.

4. Transfer the steamed chard to a serving bowl. Drizzle the garlic•lemon dressing over the top and toss to coat.

5. Serve the steamed chard warm.

The key anti•inflammatory ingredients in this recipe are:

• Swiss chard • a leafy green packed with antioxidants and anti•inflammatory compounds
• Olive oil • a healthy fat with potent anti•inflammatory properties
• Garlic • a potent anti•inflammatory food
• Lemon juice • provides vitamin C and has anti•inflammatory effects

This simple 5•ingredient steamed chard dish makes a great side or addition to any anti•inflammatory meal. Enjoy!

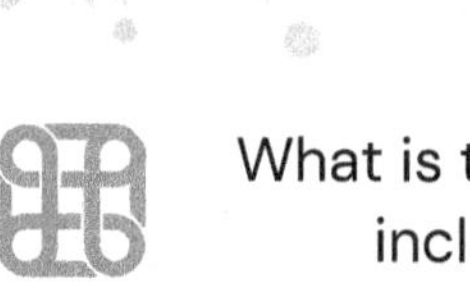

What is the total cooking time,
including prep time?

Prep Time : ________________

Cook Time : ________________

Servings   : ________________

Ingredients:

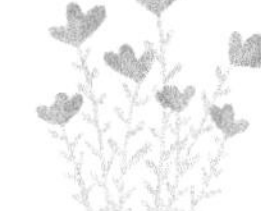

• 1 medium acorn squash, halved
and seeded
• 2 tbsp extra•virgin olive oil
• 1 tsp ground cinnamon
• 1 tsp maple syrup
• 1/4 tsp sea salt

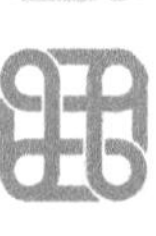
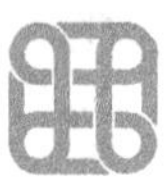
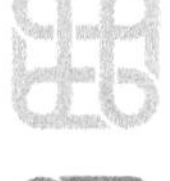
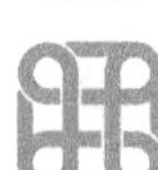

**Is the recipe easy to
follow?**

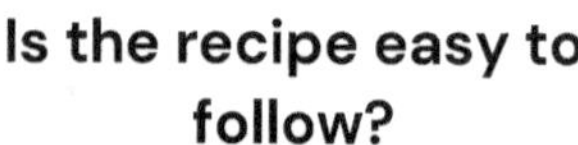

83. Grilled bitter melon with turmeric

Procedure:

1. Preheat your oven to 400°F (200°C). Line a baking sheet with parchment paper.

2. Place the acorn squash halves cut•side up on the prepared baking sheet.

3. In a small bowl, whisk together the olive oil, cinnamon, maple syrup, and sea salt.

4. Brush the cut sides of the acorn squash halves with the cinnamon•oil mixture, making sure to coat them evenly.

5. Bake for 40•50 minutes, until the squash is tender and easily pierced with a fork.

6. Remove the baked acorn squash from the oven and let cool slightly.

7. Serve the baked acorn squash warm, drizzling any remaining cinnamon•oil mixture over the top.

The key anti•inflammatory ingredients in this recipe are:

• Acorn squash • a winter squash rich in antioxidants and anti•inflammatory compounds
• Olive oil • a healthy fat with potent anti•inflammatory properties
• Cinnamon • a spice with powerful anti•inflammatory effects

This simple 5•ingredient baked acorn squash dish makes a great side or addition to any anti•inflammatory meal. Enjoy!

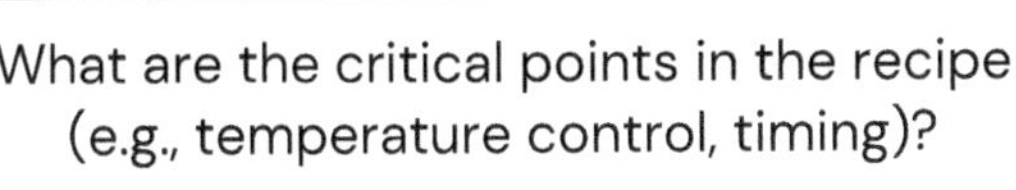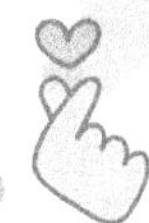

What are the critical points in the recipe (e.g., temperature control, timing)?

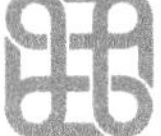
What is the total cooking time, including prep time?

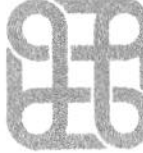
Prep Time : _______________

Cook Time : _______________

Servings   : _______________

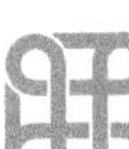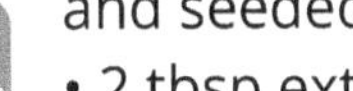

Ingredients:

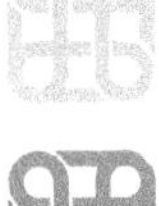
• 1 medium acorn squash, halved and seeded
• 2 tbsp extra•virgin olive oil
• 1 tsp ground cinnamon
• 1 tsp maple syrup
• 1/4 tsp sea salt

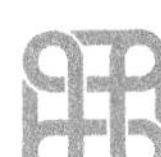
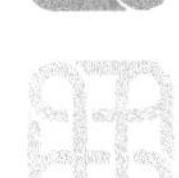
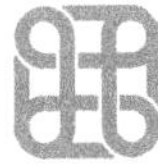
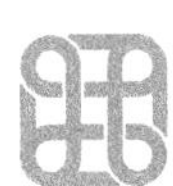

Is the recipe easy to follow?

84. Baked acorn squash with cinnamon

---

1. Preheat your oven to 400°F (200°C). Line a baking sheet with parchment paper.

2. Place the acorn squash halves cut•side up on the prepared baking sheet.

3. In a small bowl, whisk together the olive oil, cinnamon, maple syrup, and sea salt.

4. Brush the cut sides of the acorn squash halves with the cinnamon•oil mixture, making sure to coat them evenly.

5. Bake for 40•50 minutes, until the squash is tender and easily pierced with a fork.

6. Remove the baked acorn squash from the oven and let cool slightly.

7. Serve the baked acorn squash warm, drizzling any remaining cinnamon•oil mixture over the top.

The key anti•inflammatory ingredients in this recipe are:

• Acorn squash • a winter squash rich in antioxidants and anti•inflammatory compounds
• Olive oil • a healthy fat with potent anti•inflammatory properties
• Cinnamon • a spice with powerful anti•inflammatory effects

This simple 5•ingredient baked acorn squash dish makes a great side or addition to any anti•inflammatory meal. Enjoy!

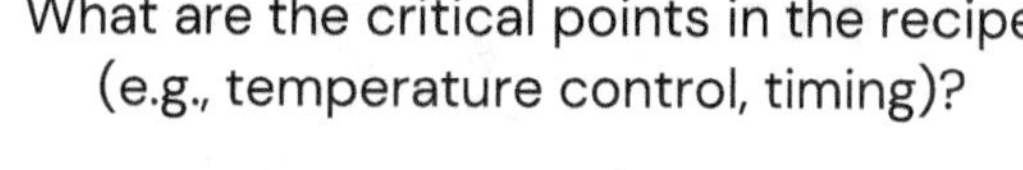

What are the critical points in the recipe (e.g., temperature control, timing)?

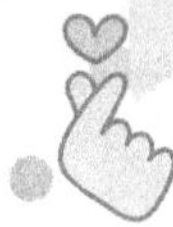

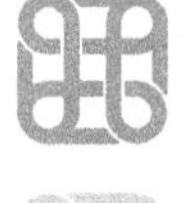

What is the total cooking time, including prep time?

Prep Time : ___________________

Cook Time : ___________________

Servings : ___________________

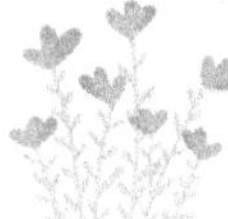

Ingredients:

- 1 lb golden beets, peeled and cut into 1•inch cubes
- 2 tbsp extra•virgin olive oil
- 1 tsp dried thyme
- 1/2 tsp sea salt
- 1/4 tsp ground black pepper

1. Preheat your oven to 400°F (200°C). Line a baking sheet with parchment paper.

2. In a large bowl, toss the golden beet cubes with the olive oil, dried thyme, sea salt, and black pepper until evenly coated.

3. Spread the seasoned beets in a single layer on the prepared baking sheet.

4. Roast for 25•30 minutes, flipping the beets halfway, until they are tender and lightly browned.

5. Remove the roasted golden beets from the oven and serve warm.

The key anti•inflammatory ingredients in this recipe are:

- Golden beets • a root vegetable rich in antioxidants and anti•inflammatory compounds
- Olive oil • a healthy fat with potent anti•inflammatory properties
- Thyme • an herb with powerful anti•inflammatory effects

This simple 5•ingredient roasted golden beets dish makes a great side or addition to any anti•inflammatory meal. Enjoy!

Is the recipe easy to follow?

85. Roasted golden beets with thyme

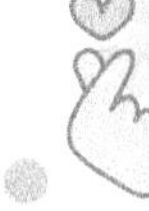

What are the critical points in the recipe (e.g., temperature control, timing)?

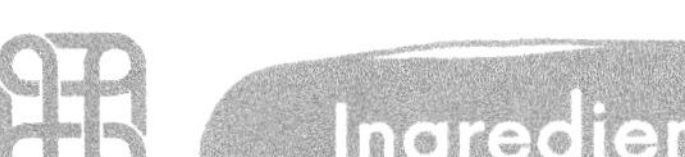

What is the total cooking time, including prep time?

Prep Time : _________________

Cook Time : _________________

Servings : _________________

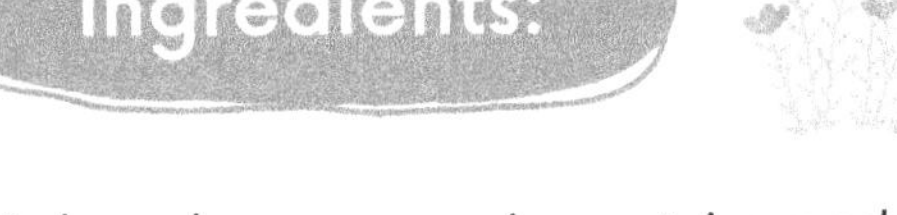

Ingredients:

• 1 bunch green onions, trimmed and halved lengthwise
• 2 tbsp extra•virgin olive oil
• 1 tbsp lemon juice
• 1/2 tsp sea salt
• 1/4 tsp ground black pepper

Is the recipe easy to follow?

86. Grilled green onions with olive oil

Procedure:

1. Preheat your grill or grill pan to medium•high heat.

2. In a small bowl, whisk together the olive oil, lemon juice, sea salt, and black pepper.

3. Brush the cut sides of the green onion halves with the olive oil mixture, making sure to coat them evenly.

4. Place the green onion halves, cut•side down, on the preheated grill. Grill for 2•3 minutes per side, until lightly charred and tender.

5. Transfer the grilled green onions to a serving platter. Drizzle any remaining olive oil mixture over the top.

6. Serve the grilled green onions warm.

The key anti•inflammatory ingredients in this recipe are:

• Green onions • contain antioxidants and anti•inflammatory compounds
• Olive oil • a healthy fat with potent anti•inflammatory properties
• Lemon juice • provides vitamin C and has anti•inflammatory effects

This simple 5•ingredient grilled green onions dish makes a great side or addition to any anti•inflammatory meal. Enjoy!

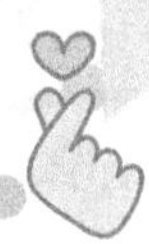

Procedure:

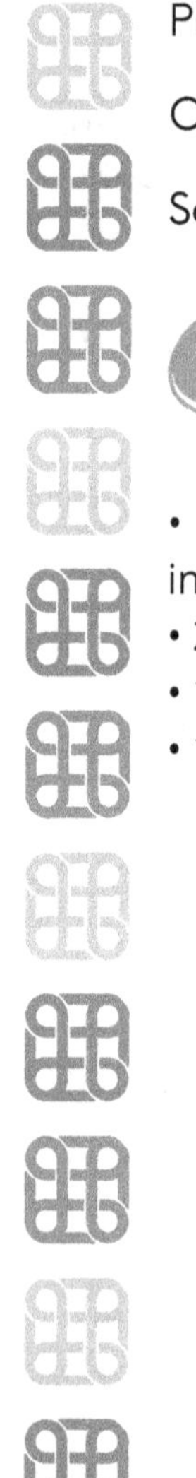

What is the total cooking time, including prep time?

Prep Time : _________________

Cook Time : _________________

Servings   : _________________

Ingredients:

• 1 lb turnips, peeled and sliced into 1/8•inch thick rounds
• 2 tbsp olive oil
• 1 tsp salt
• 1/2 tsp black pepper

Is the recipe easy to follow?

87. Baked turnip chips

1. Preheat your oven to 400°F (200°C). Line two baking sheets with parchment paper.

2. In a large bowl, toss the turnip slices with the olive oil, salt, and black pepper until evenly coated.

3. Arrange the seasoned turnip slices in a single layer on the prepared baking sheets, making sure they are not overlapping.

4. Bake for 20•25 minutes, flipping the turnip chips halfway, until they are golden brown and crispy.

5. Remove the baked turnip chips from the oven and let cool for a few minutes.

6. Serve the turnip chips warm or at room temperature.

Tips:
• Make sure to slice the turnips evenly to ensure even cooking.
• Adjust the baking time as needed, keeping a close eye on the chips to prevent burning.
• For extra crispiness, you can bake the chips in batches.

Turnips are a root vegetable that have a slightly sweet and peppery flavor when roasted. The combination of olive oil, salt, and pepper creates a delicious, savory chip.

These baked turnip chips make a great healthy snack or side dish. Enjoy their crispy texture and natural flavor!

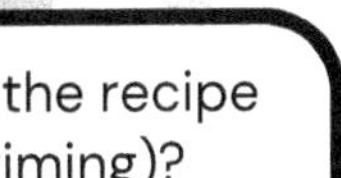

What are the critical points in the recipe (e.g., temperature control, timing)?

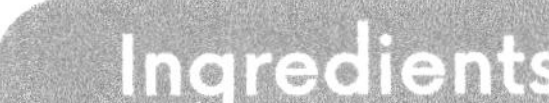

What is the total cooking time, including prep time?

Prep Time : ___________________

Cook Time : ___________________

Servings : ___________________

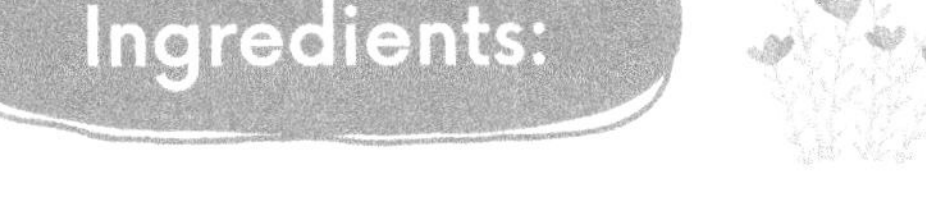
Ingredients:

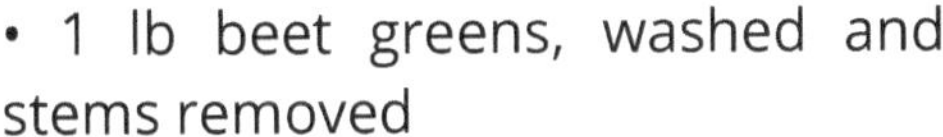

- 1 lb beet greens, washed and stems removed
- 2 tbsp extra•virgin olive oil
- 2 tbsp fresh lemon juice
- 1 tsp Dijon mustard
- 1/4 tsp sea salt

1. Fill a large pot with 1•2 inches of water and bring to a boil over high heat.

2. Add the beet greens to a steamer basket and place the basket in the pot. Cover and steam for 5•7 minutes, until the greens are tender.

3. In a small bowl, whisk together the olive oil, lemon juice, Dijon mustard, and sea salt.

4. Transfer the steamed beet greens to a serving bowl. Drizzle the lemon•mustard dressing over the top and toss to coat.

5. Serve the steamed beet greens warm.

The key anti•inflammatory ingredients in this recipe are:

- Beet greens • a leafy green packed with antioxidants and anti•inflammatory compounds
- Olive oil • a healthy fat with potent anti•inflammatory properties
- Lemon juice • provides vitamin C and has anti•inflammatory effects
- Dijon mustard • contains compounds with anti•inflammatory benefits

This simple 5•ingredient steamed beet greens dish makes a great side or addition to any anti•inflammatory meal. Enjoy!

Is the recipe easy to follow?

88. Steamed beet greens with lemon

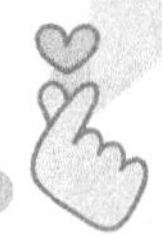

What are the critical points in the recipe (e.g., temperature control, timing)?

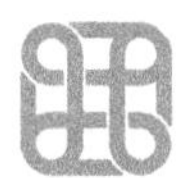
What is the total cooking time, including prep time?

Prep Time : _________________

Cook Time : _________________

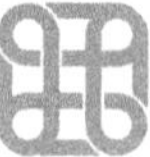
Servings : _________________

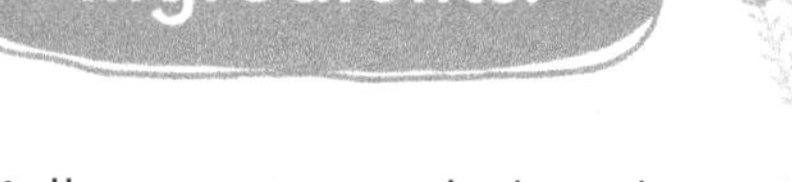

Ingredients:

- 1 lb carrots, peeled and cut into 1/2•inch thick diagonal slices
- 2 tbsp extra•virgin olive oil
- 1 tsp ground cumin
- 1 tsp lemon juice
- 1/4 tsp sea salt

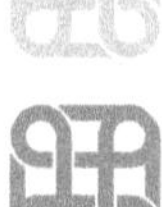 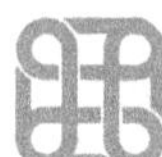 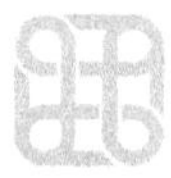 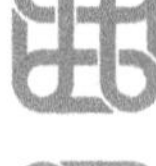 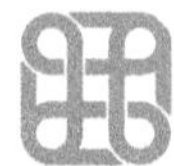

Is the recipe easy to follow?

 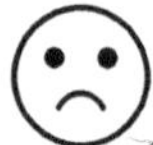

89. Grilled carrots with cumin

Procedure:

1. Preheat your grill or grill pan to medium•high heat.

2. In a large bowl, toss the carrot slices with the olive oil, ground cumin, lemon juice, and sea salt until evenly coated.

3. Arrange the seasoned carrot slices in a single layer on the preheated grill. Grill for 3•5 minutes per side, until tender and lightly charred.

4. Transfer the grilled carrots to a serving platter.

5. Serve the grilled carrots warm.

The key anti•inflammatory ingredients in this recipe are:

- Carrots • a root vegetable rich in antioxidants and anti•inflammatory compounds
- Olive oil • a healthy fat with potent anti•inflammatory properties
- Cumin • a spice with anti•inflammatory and antioxidant benefits
- Lemon juice • provides vitamin C and has anti•inflammatory effects

This simple 5•ingredient grilled carrots dish makes a great side or addition to any anti•inflammatory meal. Enjoy the smoky, spiced flavors!

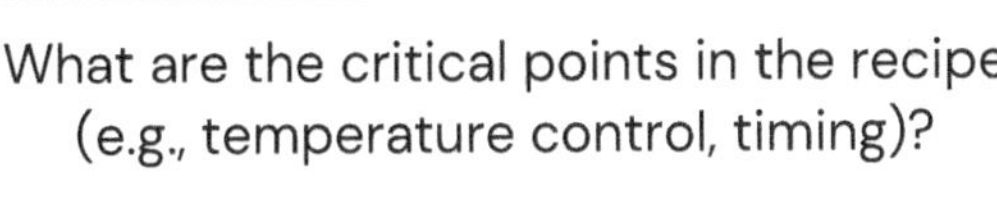

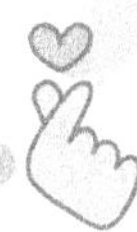

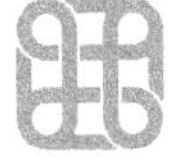

What is the total cooking time, including prep time?

Prep Time : _______________

Cook Time : _______________

Servings : _______________

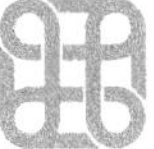
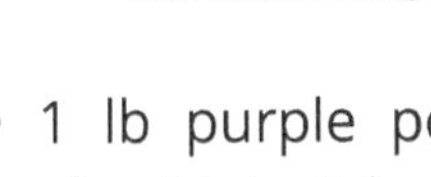

Ingredients:

- 1 lb purple potatoes, scrubbed and cut into 1•inch cubes
- 2 tbsp extra•virgin olive oil
- 1 tbsp fresh rosemary, chopped
- 1 tsp garlic powder
- 1/2 tsp sea salt

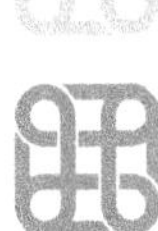
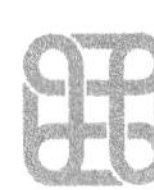
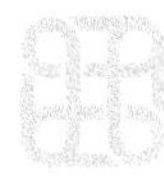
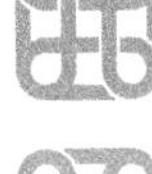
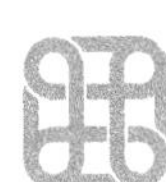

Is the recipe easy to follow?

90. Roasted purple potatoes with rosemary

1. Preheat your oven to 400°F (200°C). Line a baking sheet with parchment paper.

2. In a large bowl, toss the purple potato cubes with the olive oil, chopped rosemary, garlic powder, and sea salt until evenly coated.

3. Spread the seasoned potatoes in a single layer on the prepared baking sheet.

4. Roast for 25•30 minutes, flipping the potatoes halfway, until they are tender and lightly browned.

5. Remove the roasted purple potatoes from the oven and serve warm.

The key anti•inflammatory ingredients in this recipe are:

• Purple potatoes • a type of potato rich in antioxidants and anti•inflammatory compounds
• Olive oil • a healthy fat with potent anti•inflammatory properties
• Rosemary • an herb with powerful anti•inflammatory effects

This simple 5•ingredient roasted purple potatoes dish makes a great side or addition to any anti•inflammatory meal. Enjoy the vibrant color and earthy, herbal flavors!

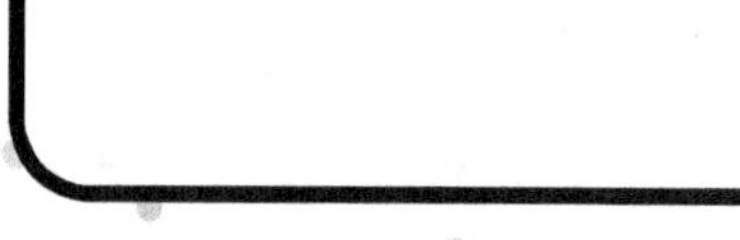

Prep Time : _______________

Cook Time : _______________

Servings   : _______________

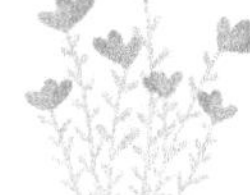

Ingredients:

• 1 delicata squash, sliced into 1/2•inch thick rings, seeds removed
• 2 tbsp extra•virgin olive oil
• 1 tsp ground cinnamon
• 1 tsp ground ginger
• 1/4 tsp sea salt

91. Baked delicata squash rings

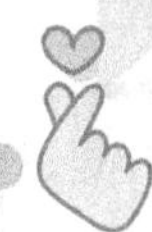

Procedure:

1. Preheat your oven to 400°F (200°C). Line a baking sheet with parchment paper.

2. In a large bowl, toss the delicata squash rings with the olive oil, cinnamon, ginger, and sea salt until evenly coated.

3. Arrange the seasoned squash rings in a single layer on the prepared baking sheet.

4. Bake for 20•25 minutes, flipping the rings halfway, until they are tender and lightly browned.

5. Remove the baked delicata squash rings from the oven and serve warm.

The key anti•inflammatory ingredients in this recipe are:

• Delicata squash • a winter squash rich in antioxidants and anti•inflammatory compounds
• Olive oil • a healthy fat with potent anti•inflammatory properties
• Cinnamon • a spice with powerful anti•inflammatory effects
• Ginger • a root with strong anti•inflammatory benefits

This simple 5•ingredient baked delicata squash rings dish makes a great side or addition to any anti•inflammatory meal. Enjoy the natural sweetness and warming spices!

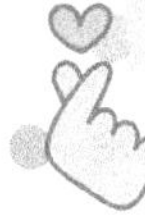

Procedure:

1. Fill a large pot with 1•2 inches of water and bring to a boil over high heat.

2. Add the kale leaves to a steamer basket and place the basket in the pot. Cover and steam for 5•7 minutes, until the kale is tender.

3. In a small bowl, whisk together the olive oil, minced garlic, lemon juice, and sea salt.

4. Transfer the steamed kale to a serving bowl. Drizzle the garlic•lemon dressing over the top and toss to coat.

5. Serve the steamed kale warm.

The key anti•inflammatory ingredients in this recipe are:

• Kale • a leafy green packed with antioxidants and anti•inflammatory compounds
• Olive oil • a healthy fat with potent anti•inflammatory properties
• Garlic • a potent anti•inflammatory food
• Lemon juice • provides vitamin C and has anti•inflammatory effects

This simple 5•ingredient steamed kale dish makes a great side or addition to any anti•inflammatory meal. Enjoy the garlicky, lemony flavor!

What is the total cooking time, including prep time?

Prep Time : _________________

Cook Time : _________________

Servings   : _________________

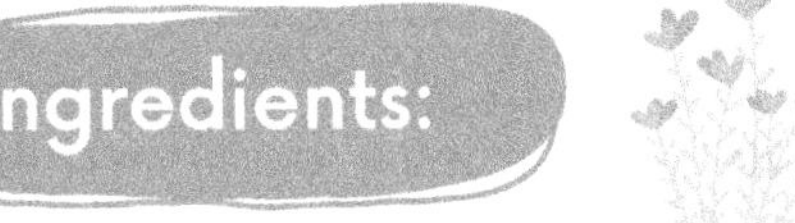

Ingredients:

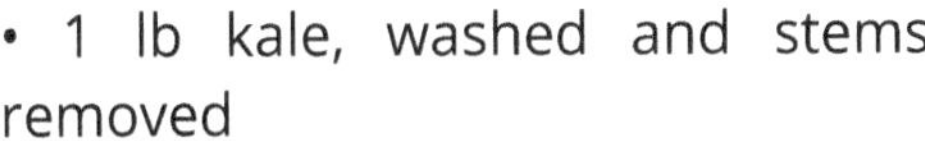

• 1 lb kale, washed and stems removed
• 2 tbsp extra•virgin olive oil
• 3 cloves garlic, minced
• 1 tbsp lemon juice
• 1/4 tsp sea salt

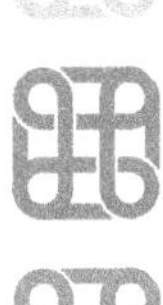
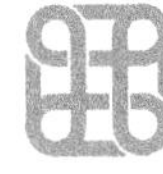
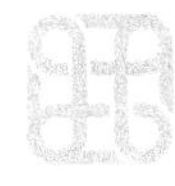
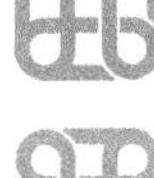
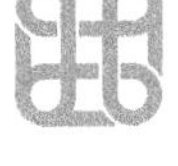

Is the recipe easy to follow?

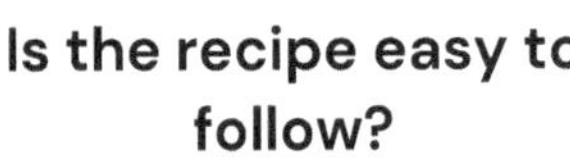

92. Steamed kale with garlic

What are the critical points in the recipe (e.g., temperature control, timing)?

What is the total cooking time, including prep time?

Prep Time : _________________

Cook Time : _________________

Servings : _________________

Ingredients:

• 2 medium zucchini, sliced lengthwise into 1/4•inch thick ribbons
• 2 tbsp extra•virgin olive oil
• 1 tbsp chopped fresh basil
• 1 tbsp chopped fresh oregano
• 1/4 tsp sea salt

Is the recipe easy to follow?

93. *Grilled zucchini ribbons with herbs*

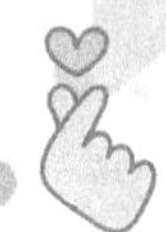

Procedure:

1. Preheat your grill or grill pan to medium•high heat.

2. In a large bowl, toss the zucchini ribbons with the olive oil, chopped basil, chopped oregano, and sea salt until evenly coated.

3. Arrange the seasoned zucchini ribbons in a single layer on the preheated grill. Grill for 2•3 minutes per side, until lightly charred and tender.

4. Transfer the grilled zucchini ribbons to a serving platter.

5. Serve the grilled zucchini ribbons warm, garnished with any remaining herb•oil mixture from the bowl.

The key anti•inflammatory ingredients in this recipe are:

• Zucchini • a summer squash rich in antioxidants and anti•inflammatory compounds
• Olive oil • a healthy fat with potent anti•inflammatory properties
• Basil and oregano • herbs with powerful anti•inflammatory effects

This simple 5•ingredient grilled zucchini ribbons dish makes a great side or addition to any anti•inflammatory meal. Enjoy the fresh, herbal flavors!

What are the critical points in the recipe (e.g., temperature control, timing)?

What is the total cooking time, including prep time?

Prep Time : _________________

Cook Time : _________________

Servings   : _________________

Ingredients:

• 1 lb taro root, peeled and sliced into 1/8•inch thick rounds
• 2 tbsp extra•virgin olive oil
• 1 tsp ground turmeric
• 1 tsp ground cumin
• 1/2 tsp sea salt

Is the recipe easy to follow?

94. Baked taro chips

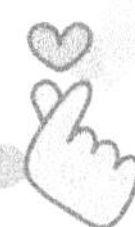

Procedure:

1. Preheat your oven to 400°F (200°C). Line two baking sheets with parchment paper.

2. In a large bowl, toss the taro slices with the olive oil, turmeric, cumin, and sea salt until evenly coated.

3. Arrange the seasoned taro slices in a single layer on the prepared baking sheets, making sure they are not overlapping.

4. Bake for 20•25 minutes, flipping the taro chips halfway, until they are golden brown and crispy.

5. Remove the baked taro chips from the oven and let cool for a few minutes.

6. Serve the taro chips warm or at room temperature.

The key anti•inflammatory ingredients in this recipe are:

• Taro root • a root vegetable rich in antioxidants and anti•inflammatory compounds
• Olive oil • a healthy fat with potent anti•inflammatory properties
• Turmeric • a spice with powerful anti•inflammatory effects
• Cumin • a spice with anti•inflammatory and antioxidant benefits

These baked taro chips make a great healthy snack or side dish that supports an anti•inflammatory diet. Enjoy their crispy texture and flavorful spices!

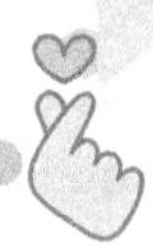

What are the critical points in the recipe (e.g., temperature control, timing)?

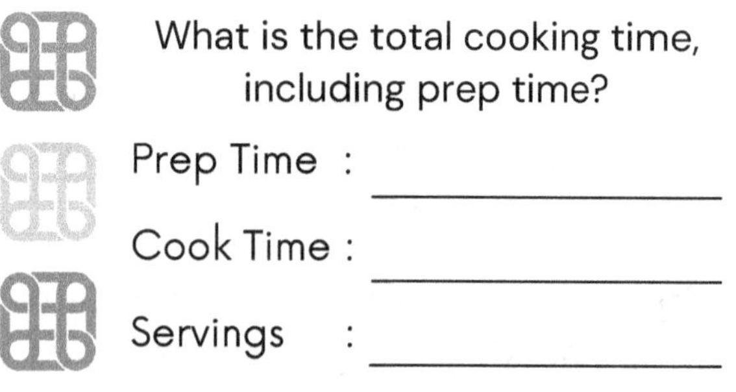

What is the total cooking time, including prep time?

Prep Time : _______________

Cook Time : _______________

Servings   : _______________

Ingredients:

• 1 lb parsnips, peeled and cut into 1•inch pieces
• 2 tbsp extra•virgin olive oil
• 1 tsp dried thyme
• 1 tsp maple syrup
• 1/4 tsp sea salt

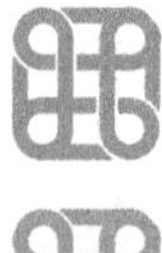
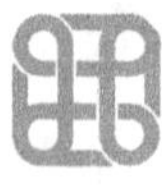
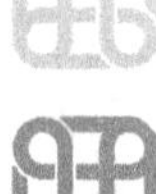
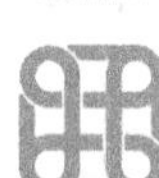
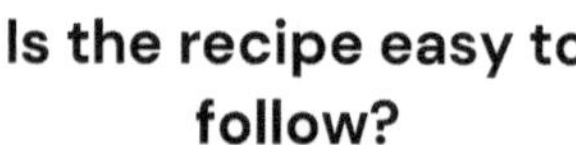

Is the recipe easy to follow?

95. Roasted parsnips with thyme

Procedure:

1. Preheat your oven to 400°F (200°C). Line a baking sheet with parchment paper.

2. In a large bowl, toss the parsnip pieces with the olive oil, dried thyme, maple syrup, and sea salt until evenly coated.

3. Spread the seasoned parsnips in a single layer on the prepared baking sheet.

4. Roast for 25•30 minutes, flipping the parsnips halfway, until they are tender and lightly browned.

5. Remove the roasted parsnips from the oven and serve warm.

The key anti•inflammatory ingredients in this recipe are:

• Parsnips • a root vegetable rich in antioxidants and anti•inflammatory compounds
• Olive oil • a healthy fat with potent anti•inflammatory properties
• Thyme • an herb with powerful anti•inflammatory effects

This simple 5•ingredient roasted parsnips dish makes a great side or addition to any anti•inflammatory meal. Enjoy the natural sweetness and earthy, herbal flavors!

Procedure:

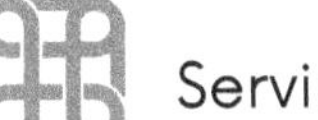

What is the total cooking time, including prep time?

Prep Time : _________________

Cook Time : _________________

Servings   : _________________

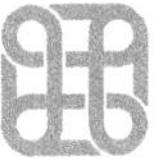

Ingredients:

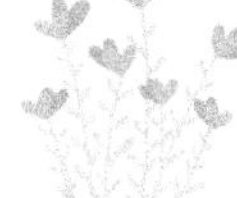

- 1 lb baby bok choy, halved lengthwise
- 2 tbsp sesame oil
- 1 tbsp rice vinegar
- 1 tsp toasted sesame seeds
- 1/4 tsp sea salt

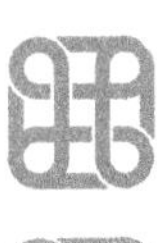
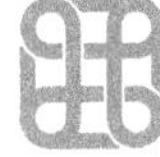
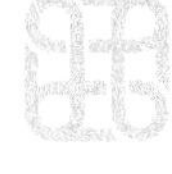
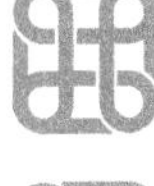
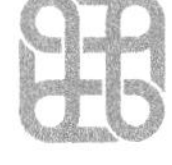

1. Preheat your grill or grill pan to medium•high heat.

2. In a large bowl, toss the baby bok choy halves with the sesame oil, rice vinegar, toasted sesame seeds, and sea salt until evenly coated.

3. Arrange the seasoned bok choy halves, cut•side down, on the preheated grill. Grill for 2•3 minutes per side, until lightly charred and tender.

4. Transfer the grilled baby bok choy to a serving platter.

5. Serve the grilled bok choy warm, drizzling any remaining sesame•vinegar mixture over the top.

The key anti•inflammatory ingredients in this recipe are:

• Baby bok choy • a cruciferous vegetable rich in antioxidants and anti•inflammatory compounds
• Sesame oil • a healthy fat with anti•inflammatory properties
• Rice vinegar • contains acetic acid with anti•inflammatory effects

This simple 5•ingredient grilled baby bok choy dish makes a great side or addition to any anti•inflammatory meal. Enjoy the smoky, nutty flavors!

Is the recipe easy to follow?

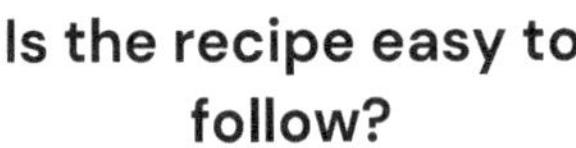

96. Grilled baby bok choy

What are the critical points in the recipe (e.g., temperature control, timing)?

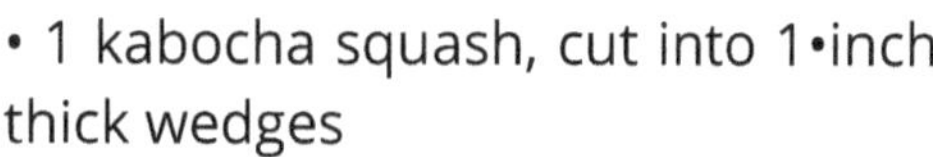

What is the total cooking time, including prep time?

Prep Time : ________________

Cook Time : ________________

Servings : ________________

Ingredients:

• 1 kabocha squash, cut into 1•inch thick wedges
• 2 tbsp olive oil
• 1 tsp salt
• 1/2 tsp black pepper
• 1/2 tsp garlic powder (optional)
• 1/2 tsp paprika (optional)

Is the recipe easy to follow?

97. Baked kabocha squash wedges

Procedure:

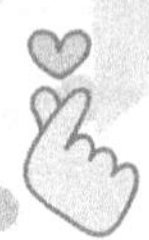

1. Preheat your oven to 400°F (200°C).

2. Wash the kabocha squash and cut it in half lengthwise. Scoop out the seeds and cut each half into 1•inch thick wedges.

3. In a large bowl, toss the squash wedges with the olive oil, salt, black pepper, and any other desired seasonings like garlic powder or paprika.

4. Arrange the seasoned squash wedges in a single layer on a baking sheet lined with parchment paper or a silicone baking mat.

5. Bake for 25•30 minutes, flipping the wedges halfway through, until the squash is tender and lightly browned on the edges.

6. Serve the baked kabocha squash wedges hot, as a side dish or snack. They pair well with proteins, salads, or can be enjoyed on their own.

Enjoy the sweet, nutty flavor and creamy texture of the roasted kabocha squash!

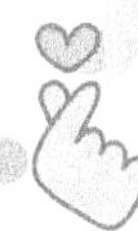

What are the critical points in the recipe (e.g., temperature control, timing)?

What is the total cooking time, including prep time?

Prep Time : _______________

Cook Time : _______________

Servings   : _______________

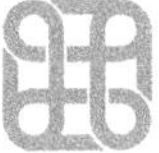

Ingredients:

- 1 lb watercress, washed and stems removed
- 2 tbsp extra•virgin olive oil
- 1 tbsp freshly grated ginger
- 1 tbsp rice vinegar
- 1/4 tsp sea salt

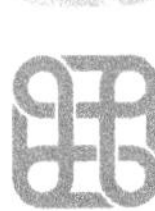
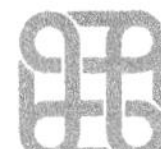

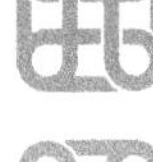
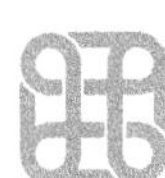

Is the recipe easy to follow?

98. Steamed watercress with ginger

1. Fill a large pot with 1•2 inches of water and bring to a boil over high heat.

2. Add the watercress to a steamer basket and place the basket in the pot. Cover and steam for 3•5 minutes, until the watercress is tender.

3. In a small bowl, whisk together the olive oil, grated ginger, rice vinegar, and sea salt.

4. Transfer the steamed watercress to a serving bowl. Drizzle the ginger•vinegar dressing over the top and toss to coat.

5. Serve the steamed watercress warm.

The key anti•inflammatory ingredients in this recipe are:

- Watercress • a leafy green packed with antioxidants and anti•inflammatory compounds
- Olive oil • a healthy fat with potent anti•inflammatory properties
- Ginger • a root with strong anti•inflammatory benefits
- Rice vinegar • contains acetic acid with anti•inflammatory effects

This simple 5•ingredient steamed watercress dish makes a great side or addition to any anti•inflammatory meal. Enjoy the bright, gingery flavor!

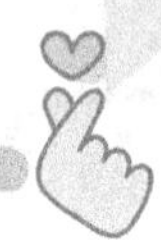

What are the critical points in the recipe (e.g., temperature control, timing)?

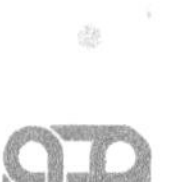

What is the total cooking time, including prep time?

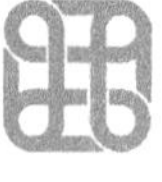

Prep Time : ________________

Cook Time : ________________

Servings   : ________________

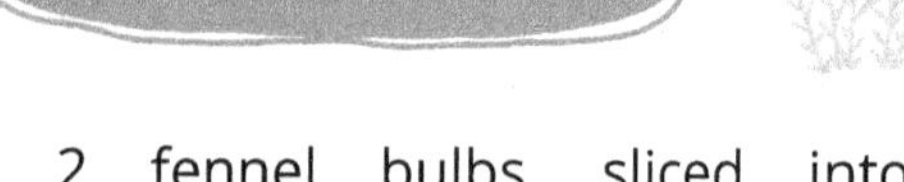

Ingredients:

- 2 fennel bulbs, sliced into 1/2•inch thick wedges
- 2 tbsp olive oil
- 1 tsp lemon juice
- 1/2 tsp salt
- 1/4 tsp black pepper

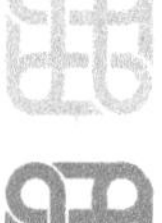
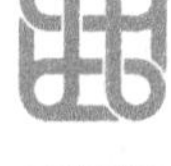
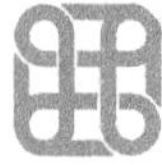
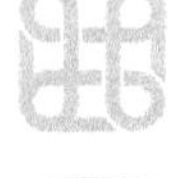
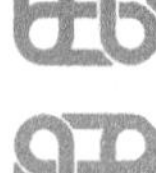
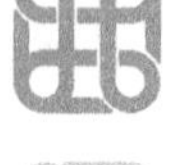
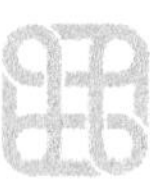

Is the recipe easy to follow?

99. Grilled fennel bulbs

1. Preheat your grill or grill pan to medium•high heat.

2. In a large bowl, toss the fennel wedges with the olive oil, lemon juice, salt, and black pepper until evenly coated.

3. Arrange the seasoned fennel wedges on the preheated grill or grill pan. Grill for 4•5 minutes per side, or until tender and lightly charred.

4. Transfer the grilled fennel wedges to a serving plate.

5. Serve the grilled fennel warm, as a side dish. It pairs well with grilled meats, fish, or can be enjoyed on its own.

The key anti•inflammatory ingredients in this recipe are:

- Fennel • Contains anti•inflammatory compounds like anethole and quercetin.
- Olive oil • Rich in monounsaturated fats and polyphenols with anti•inflammatory properties.
- Lemon juice • Provides vitamin C, which has antioxidant and anti•inflammatory effects.
- Black pepper • Contains piperine, which has been shown to have anti•inflammatory benefits.

This simple grilled fennel dish makes a great addition to an anti•inflammatory diet. Enjoy!

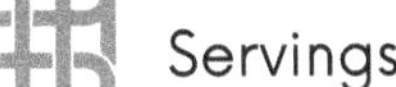

What is the total cooking time, including prep time?

Prep Time : ________________

Cook Time : ________________

Servings   : ________________

Ingredients:

- 2 lbs rutabaga, peeled and cut into 1•inch cubes
- 2 tbsp olive oil
- 1 tsp ground cumin
- 1/2 tsp salt
- 1/4 tsp black pepper

Is the recipe easy to follow?

100. Roasted rutabaga with olive oil

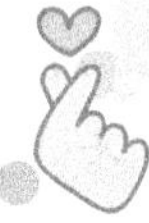

Procedure:

1. Preheat your oven to 400°F (200°C).

2. In a large bowl, toss the cubed rutabaga with the olive oil, cumin, salt, and black pepper until the rutabaga is evenly coated.

3. Spread the seasoned rutabaga cubes in a single layer on a baking sheet lined with parchment paper.

4. Roast the rutabaga for 25•30 minutes, flipping halfway through, until tender and lightly browned.

5. Transfer the roasted rutabaga to a serving dish and serve hot.

The key anti•inflammatory ingredients in this recipe are:

- Rutabaga • Contains glucosinolates and other compounds with anti•inflammatory properties.
- Olive oil • Rich in monounsaturated fats and polyphenols with anti•inflammatory effects.
- Cumin • Contains compounds like cuminaldehyde that have been shown to have anti•inflammatory benefits.
- Black pepper • Contains piperine, which has been demonstrated to have anti•inflammatory effects.

This simple roasted rutabaga dish makes a great side for an anti•inflammatory diet. The combination of flavors and nutrients from the ingredients provides a delicious and healthy option.

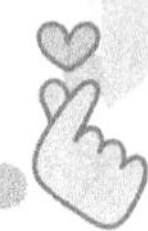

What are the critical points in the recipe (e.g., temperature control, timing)?

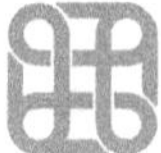 What is the total cooking time, including prep time?

Prep Time : _______________

Cook Time : _______________

Servings : _______________

Ingredients:

• 1 lb lotus root, peeled and sliced into 1/8•inch thick rounds
• 2 tbsp olive oil
• 1 tsp ground turmeric
• 1/2 tsp salt
• 1/4 tsp black pepper

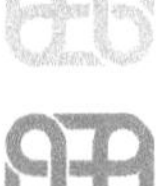 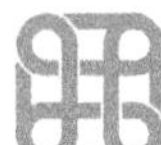 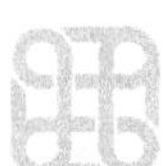 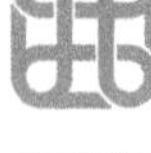 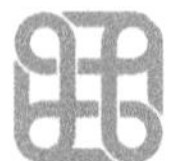

Is the recipe easy to follow?

101. Baked lotus root chips

1. Preheat your oven to 400°F (200°C). Line a baking sheet with parchment paper.

2. In a large bowl, toss the lotus root slices with the olive oil, turmeric, salt, and black pepper until the slices are evenly coated.

3. Arrange the seasoned lotus root slices in a single layer on the prepared baking sheet.

4. Bake for 18•22 minutes, flipping the slices halfway through, until they are crispy and lightly browned.

5. Remove the baked lotus root chips from the oven and let them cool slightly before serving.

The key anti•inflammatory ingredients in this recipe are:

• Lotus root • Contains antioxidants and anti•inflammatory compounds like vitamin C and quercetin.
• Olive oil • Rich in monounsaturated fats and polyphenols with anti•inflammatory effects.
• Turmeric • Contains the active compound curcumin, which has potent anti•inflammatory properties.
• Black pepper • Contains piperine, which has been shown to enhance the bioavailability of curcumin and other anti•inflammatory compounds.

These baked lotus root chips make a delicious and healthy snack or side dish that supports an anti•inflammatory diet. Enjoy the crispy texture and earthy, slightly sweet flavor of the lotus root.

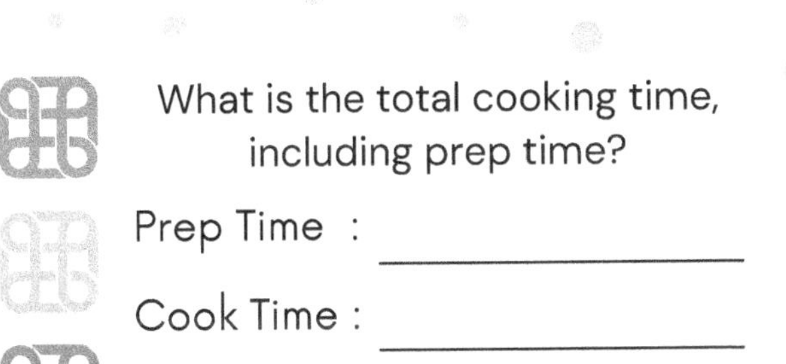

What is the total cooking time, including prep time?

Prep Time : _______________

Cook Time : _______________

Servings   : _______________

Ingredients:

- 1 lb broccoli rabe, washed and trimmed
- 2 tbsp olive oil
- 3 cloves garlic, minced
- 1/2 tsp salt
- 1/4 tsp red pepper flakes (optional)

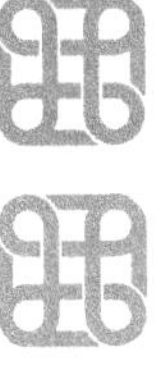
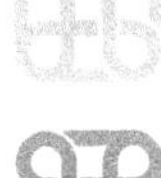
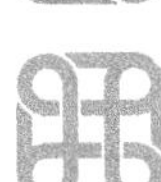

Is the recipe easy to follow?

102. Steamed broccoli rabe with garlic

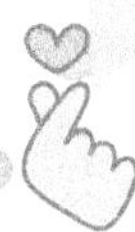

Procedure:

1. Fill a large pot with 1·2 inches of water and bring it to a boil.

2. Place the broccoli rabe in a steamer basket and steam for 3·5 minutes, or until the stems are tender but still crisp.

3. In a small skillet, heat the olive oil over medium heat. Add the minced garlic and sauté for 1·2 minutes, until fragrant.

4. Transfer the steamed broccoli rabe to a serving bowl. Drizzle the garlic·infused olive oil over the greens and toss to coat.

5. Season the steamed broccoli rabe with salt and red pepper flakes (if using).

6. Serve the steamed broccoli rabe with garlic warm.

The broccoli rabe provides a slightly bitter, peppery flavor that pairs well with the aromatic garlic. The olive oil helps to coat and lightly dress the greens, while the salt and optional red pepper flakes add depth of flavor.

Broccoli rabe is a nutrient·dense green that is rich in vitamins, minerals, and antioxidants. The garlic also provides anti·inflammatory benefits, making this a great side dish to support overall health.

This simple steamed broccoli rabe with garlic makes a wonderful accompaniment to grilled or roasted proteins, or can be enjoyed on its own as a healthy vegetable side dish.

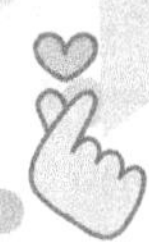

Procedure:

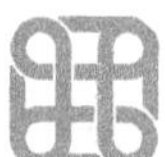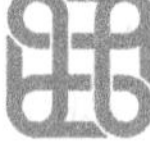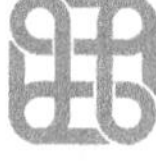 What is the total cooking time, including prep time?

Prep Time : ___________

Cook Time : ___________

Servings : ___________

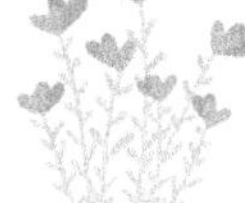

Ingredients:

• 4 heads Belgian endive, halved lengthwise
• 2 tbsp olive oil
• 2 tbsp balsamic vinegar
• 1 tsp honey
• 1/4 tsp salt

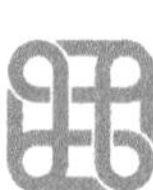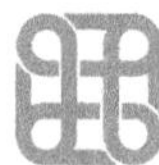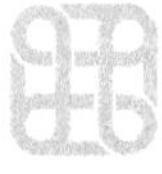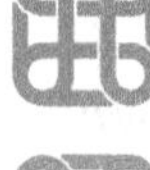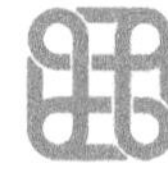

1. Preheat your grill or grill pan to medium•high heat.

2. In a small bowl, whisk together the olive oil, balsamic vinegar, honey, and salt.

3. Brush or drizzle the balsamic vinaigrette over the cut sides of the endive halves, making sure to coat them evenly.

4. Grill the endive halves for 2•3 minutes per side, or until they are lightly charred and slightly softened.

5. Transfer the grilled Belgian endive to a serving plate.

The key anti•inflammatory ingredients in this recipe are:

• Belgian endive • A type of chicory that contains anti•inflammatory compounds like vitamin K and polyphenols.
• Olive oil • Provides monounsaturated fats and polyphenols with anti•inflammatory effects.
• Balsamic vinegar • Contains acetic acid and polyphenols that may have anti•inflammatory properties.
• Honey • Provides antioxidants and may have mild anti•inflammatory benefits.

The grilling process helps to balance the natural bitterness of the Belgian endive, while the sweet and tangy balsamic vinaigrette adds a delicious contrast of flavors.

These grilled Belgian endive with balsamic make a great side dish for grilled or roasted proteins, or can be enjoyed on their own as part of an anti•inflammatory meal. The combination of flavors and nutrients from the ingredients provides a healthy and flavorful option.

Is the recipe easy to follow?

103. Grilled Belgian endive with balsamic

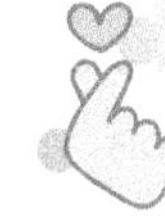

Procedure:

What is the total cooking time, including prep time?

Prep Time : ______________

Cook Time : ______________

Servings : ______________

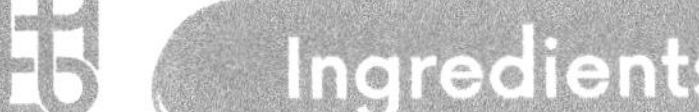

Ingredients:

- 1 medium butternut squash, peeled, seeded, and spiralized into noodles
- 2 tbsp olive oil
- 1 tsp dried thyme
- 1/2 tsp salt
- 1/4 tsp black pepper

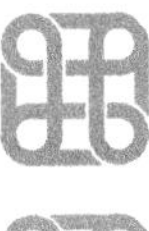 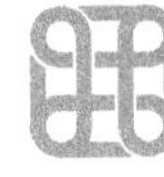 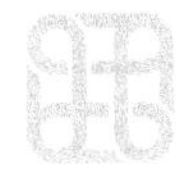 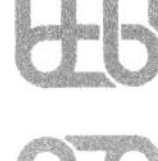 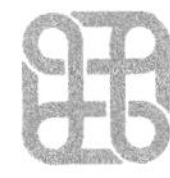

Is the recipe easy to follow?

104. Baked butternut squash noodles

1. Preheat your oven to 400°F (200°C). Line a baking sheet with parchment paper.

2. In a large bowl, toss the butternut squash noodles with the olive oil, dried thyme, salt, and black pepper until the noodles are evenly coated.

3. Spread the seasoned butternut squash noodles in a single layer on the prepared baking sheet.

4. Bake for 18•22 minutes, flipping the noodles halfway through, until they are tender and lightly browned.

5. Remove the baked butternut squash noodles from the oven and transfer them to a serving dish.

The baked butternut squash noodles have a delicate, slightly sweet flavor and a tender, pasta•like texture. The olive oil, thyme, salt, and pepper help to enhance the natural flavors of the squash.

Butternut squash is a nutrient•dense vegetable that is rich in vitamins, minerals, and antioxidants. Spiralizing the squash into noodles creates a fun and healthy alternative to traditional pasta.

These baked butternut squash noodles make a great side dish or can be used as a base for a variety of toppings and sauces. They pair well with grilled or roasted proteins, or can be enjoyed on their own as a satisfying and nutritious meal.

Enjoy the delicious and versatile baked butternut squash noodles!

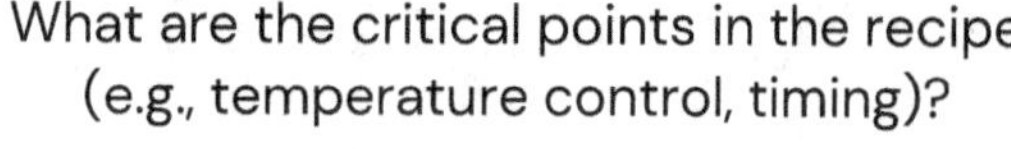
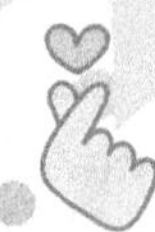

What are the critical points in the recipe (e.g., temperature control, timing)?

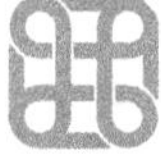

What is the total cooking time, including prep time?

Prep Time : ________________

Cook Time : ________________

Servings   : ________________

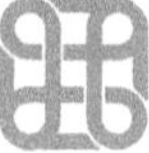

Ingredients:

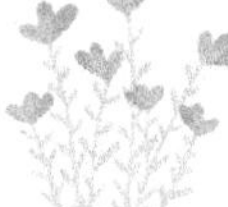

- 1 lb sunchokes, scrubbed and cut into 1•inch pieces
- 2 tbsp olive oil
- 2 tsp chopped fresh rosemary
- 1 tsp salt
- 1/2 tsp black pepper

Is the recipe easy to follow?

105. Roasted sunchokes with rosemary

Procedure:

1. Preheat your oven to 400°F (200°C). Line a baking sheet with parchment paper.

2. In a large bowl, toss the sunchoke pieces with the olive oil, chopped rosemary, salt, and black pepper until the sunchokes are evenly coated.

3. Spread the seasoned sunchoke pieces in a single layer on the prepared baking sheet.

4. Roast the sunchokes for 25•30 minutes, flipping them halfway through, until they are tender and lightly browned.

5. Remove the roasted sunchokes from the oven and transfer them to a serving dish.

6. Serve the roasted sunchokes with rosemary warm, as a side dish.

The earthy, nutty flavor of the sunchokes pairs beautifully with the fragrant rosemary in this simple roasted vegetable dish. The olive oil, salt, and pepper help to enhance the natural flavors of the sunchokes.

Sunchokes are a unique root vegetable that are rich in fiber, vitamins, and minerals. Roasting them brings out their natural sweetness and creates a creamy, tender texture.

This roasted sunchoke with rosemary recipe makes a great side dish to accompany roasted meats, fish, or as part of a vegetarian meal. Enjoy the delicious combination of flavors!

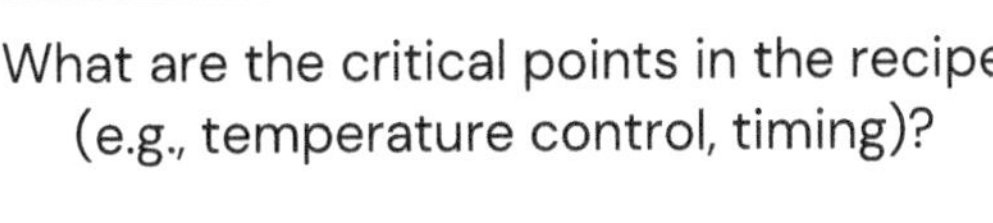

What are the critical points in the recipe (e.g., temperature control, timing)?

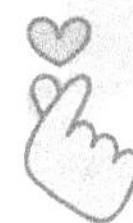

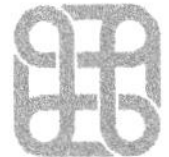

What is the total cooking time, including prep time?

Prep Time : ___________________

Cook Time : ___________________

Servings   : ___________________

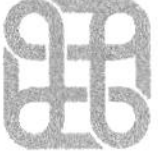

Ingredients:

- 1 head radicchio, cut into 1•inch thick wedges
- 2 tbsp olive oil
- 1 tbsp balsamic vinegar
- 1 tsp honey
- 1/4 tsp salt

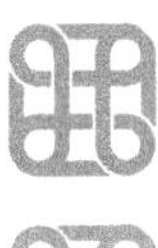
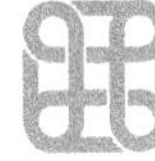
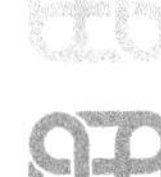
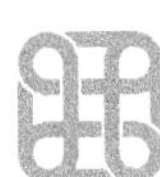

Is the recipe easy to follow?

106. Grilled radicchio wedges

1. Preheat your grill or grill pan to medium•high heat.

2. In a small bowl, whisk together the olive oil, balsamic vinegar, honey, and salt.

3. Brush or drizzle the vinaigrette over the radicchio wedges, making sure to coat them evenly on both sides.

4. Grill the radicchio wedges for 2•3 minutes per side, or until they are lightly charred and slightly softened.

5. Transfer the grilled radicchio wedges to a serving plate.

The key anti•inflammatory ingredients in this recipe are:

- Radicchio • A type of chicory that contains anti•inflammatory compounds like vitamin K and polyphenols.
- Olive oil • Provides monounsaturated fats and polyphenols with anti•inflammatory effects.
- Balsamic vinegar • Contains acetic acid and polyphenols that may have anti•inflammatory properties.
- Honey • Provides antioxidants and may have mild anti•inflammatory benefits.

The grilling process helps to balance the natural bitterness of the radicchio, while the sweet and tangy vinaigrette adds a delicious contrast of flavors.

These grilled radicchio wedges make a great side dish for grilled or roasted proteins, or can be enjoyed on their own as part of an anti•inflammatory meal. The combination of flavors and nutrients from the ingredients provides a healthy and flavorful option.

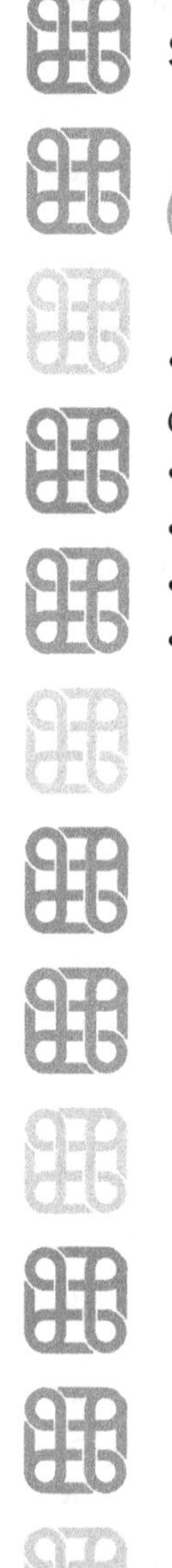

What are the critical points in the recipe (e.g., temperature control, timing)?

What is the total cooking time, including prep time?

Prep Time : _______________

Cook Time : _______________

Servings : _______________

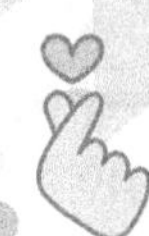

Ingredients:

• 1 lb yuca (cassava), peeled and cut into 1/2•inch thick fry shapes
• 2 tbsp olive oil
• 1 tsp ground cumin
• 1/2 tsp salt
• 1/4 tsp cayenne pepper

Is the recipe easy to follow?

☺ ☹

107. Baked yuca fries

Procedure:

1. Preheat your oven to 400°F (200°C). Line a baking sheet with parchment paper.

2. In a large bowl, toss the yuca fries with the olive oil, cumin, salt, and cayenne pepper until the fries are evenly coated.

3. Arrange the seasoned yuca fries in a single layer on the prepared baking sheet.

4. Bake for 25•30 minutes, flipping the fries halfway through, until they are golden brown and crispy.

5. Remove the baked yuca fries from the oven and let them cool slightly before serving.

The key anti•inflammatory ingredients in this recipe are:

• Yuca (cassava) • Contains anti•inflammatory compounds like vitamin C, manganese, and phenolic antioxidants.
• Olive oil • Rich in monounsaturated fats and polyphenols with anti•inflammatory effects.
• Cumin • Contains compounds like cuminaldehyde that have been shown to have anti•inflammatory benefits.
• Cayenne pepper • Contains capsaicin, which has been demonstrated to have potent anti•inflammatory properties.

These baked yuca fries make a delicious and healthy alternative to traditional french fries. The combination of flavors and nutrients from the ingredients provides an anti•inflammatory boost to this tasty snack or side dish.

What are the critical points in the recipe (e.g., temperature control, timing)?

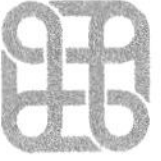

What is the total cooking time, including prep time?

Prep Time : _______________

Cook Time : _______________

Servings : _______________

Ingredients:

• 1 head napa cabbage, shredded or thinly sliced
• 2 tbsp sesame oil
• 2 tsp grated fresh ginger
• 1 tsp rice vinegar
• 1/4 tsp salt

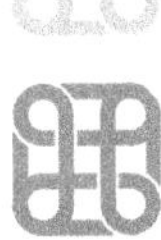
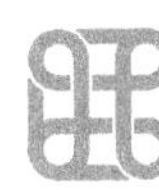
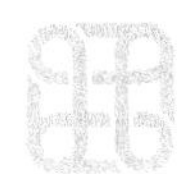
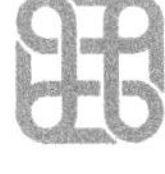
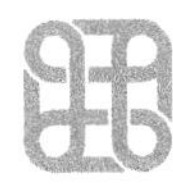

Is the recipe easy to follow?

108. Steamed napa cabbage with ginger

1. Fill a large pot with 1•2 inches of water and bring it to a boil.

2. Place the shredded or sliced napa cabbage in a steamer basket and steam for 3•5 minutes, or until the cabbage is tender but still crisp.

3. In a small bowl, whisk together the sesame oil, grated ginger, rice vinegar, and salt.

4. Transfer the steamed napa cabbage to a serving dish and drizzle the ginger•sesame dressing over the top. Toss gently to coat.

5. Serve the steamed napa cabbage with ginger warm or at room temperature.

The key anti•inflammatory ingredients in this recipe are:

• Napa cabbage • Contains glucosinolates and other anti•inflammatory compounds.
• Sesame oil • Provides anti•inflammatory omega•6 fatty acids.
• Ginger • Contains the active compound gingerol, which has potent anti•inflammatory properties.
• Rice vinegar • Helps to balance the flavors and may have mild anti•inflammatory effects.

This simple steamed napa cabbage dish with ginger makes a great side for an anti•inflammatory diet. The bright, slightly tangy flavors of the ginger•sesame dressing complement the tender, sweet napa cabbage perfectly.

Enjoy this steamed napa cabbage as a side to grilled or roasted proteins, or as part of a larger anti•inflammatory meal.

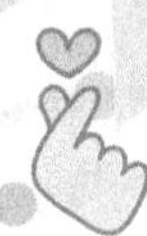

What are the critical points in the recipe (e.g., temperature control, timing)?

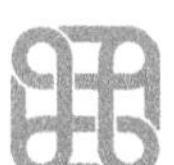 What is the total cooking time, including prep time?

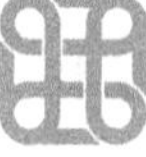 Prep Time : _________________

Cook Time : _________________

Servings : _________________

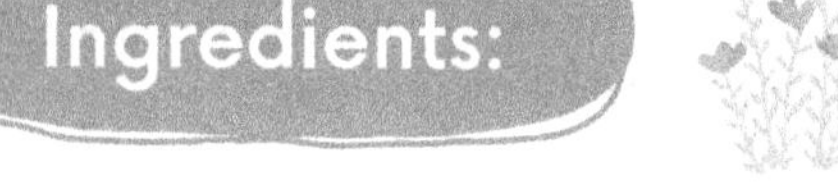

Ingredients:

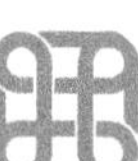
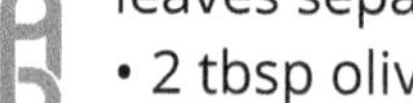

• 1 head escarole, washed and leaves separated
• 2 tbsp olive oil
• 1 tbsp lemon juice
• 1 tsp Dijon mustard
• 1/4 tsp salt

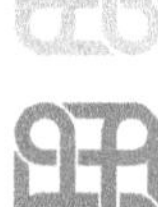
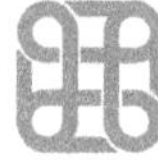
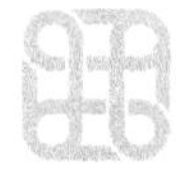
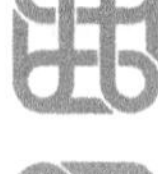
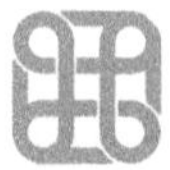

Is the recipe easy to follow?

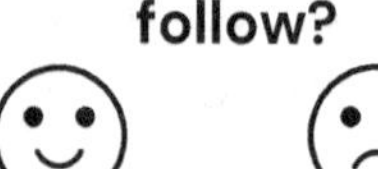

109. Grilled escarole

Procedure:

1. Preheat your grill or grill pan to medium•high heat.

2. In a large bowl, whisk together the olive oil, lemon juice, Dijon mustard, and salt.

3. Add the escarole leaves to the bowl and toss gently to coat them evenly with the dressing.

4. Grill the escarole leaves for 2•3 minutes per side, or until they are lightly charred and wilted.

5. Transfer the grilled escarole to a serving plate or bowl.

The key anti•inflammatory ingredients in this recipe are:

• Escarole • A leafy green that contains anti•inflammatory compounds like vitamin K, folate, and polyphenols.
• Olive oil • Provides monounsaturated fats and polyphenols with anti•inflammatory effects.
• Lemon juice • Contains vitamin C, which has antioxidant and anti•inflammatory properties.
• Dijon mustard • May have mild anti•inflammatory benefits due to its phytochemical content.

The grilling process helps to enhance the natural bitterness of the escarole, while the simple dressing of olive oil, lemon, and mustard balances the flavors and provides an anti•inflammatory boost.

This grilled escarole dish makes a great side for grilled or roasted proteins, or can be enjoyed on its own as a healthy, anti•inflammatory•friendly vegetable.

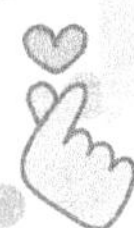

What is the total cooking time,
including prep time?

Prep Time : _______________

Cook Time : _______________

Servings   : _______________

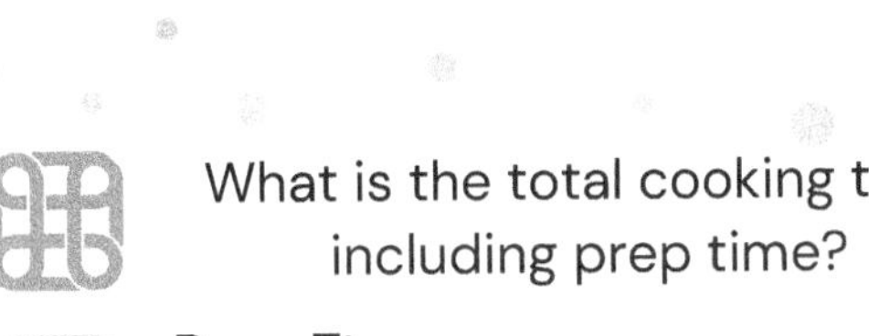

Ingredients:

- 1 lb celeriac (celery root), peeled and cut into 1·inch cubes
- 2 tbsp olive oil
- 2 tsp fresh thyme leaves, chopped
- 1 tsp salt
- 1/2 tsp black pepper

Is the recipe easy to follow?

110. Roasted celeriac with thyme

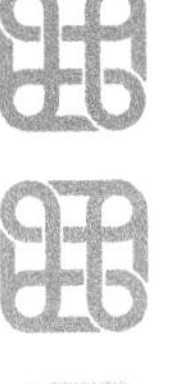
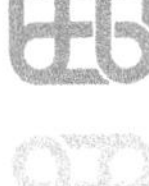
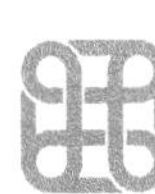
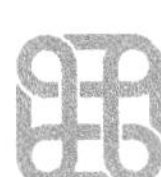

1. Preheat your oven to 400°F (200°C). Line a baking sheet with parchment paper.

2. In a large bowl, toss the celeriac cubes with the olive oil, chopped thyme, salt, and black pepper until the celeriac is evenly coated.

3. Spread the seasoned celeriac cubes in a single layer on the prepared baking sheet.

4. Roast the celeriac for 25·30 minutes, flipping halfway through, until it is tender and lightly browned.

5. Remove the roasted celeriac from the oven and transfer it to a serving dish.

6. Serve the roasted celeriac warm, garnished with additional fresh thyme leaves if desired.

The earthy, slightly nutty flavor of the celeriac pairs beautifully with the fragrant thyme in this simple roasted vegetable dish. The olive oil, salt, and pepper help to enhance the natural flavors of the celeriac.

Celeriac is a versatile root vegetable that is rich in fiber, vitamins, and minerals. Roasting it brings out its natural sweetness and creates a creamy, tender texture.

This roasted celeriac with thyme makes a great side dish to accompany roasted meats, fish, or as part of a vegetarian meal. Enjoy the delicious combination of flavors!

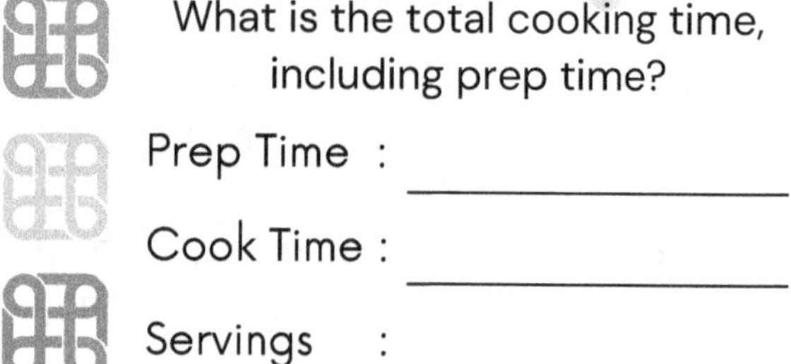

What is the total cooking time, including prep time?

Prep Time : _______________

Cook Time : _______________

Servings   : _______________

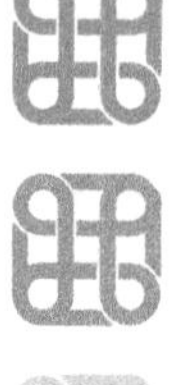

Ingredients:

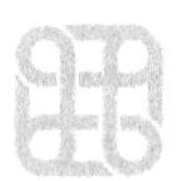

• 2 green plantains, peeled and sliced into 1/8•inch thick rounds
• 2 tbsp olive oil
• 1 tsp ground turmeric
• 1/2 tsp salt
• 1/4 tsp black pepper

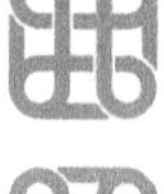
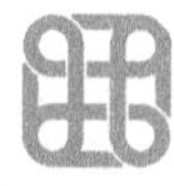
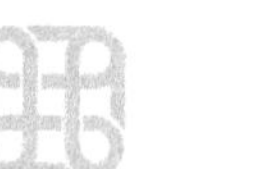

Is the recipe easy to follow?

111. Baked plantain chips

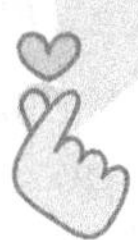

Procedure:

1. Preheat your oven to 400°F (200°C). Line a baking sheet with parchment paper.

2. In a large bowl, toss the plantain slices with the olive oil, turmeric, salt, and black pepper until the slices are evenly coated.

3. Arrange the seasoned plantain slices in a single layer on the prepared baking sheet.

4. Bake for 18•22 minutes, flipping the slices halfway through, until they are crispy and lightly browned.

5. Remove the baked plantain chips from the oven and let them cool slightly before serving.

The key anti•inflammatory ingredients in this recipe are:

• Green plantains • Contain resistant starch and other compounds with anti•inflammatory properties.
• Olive oil • Rich in monounsaturated fats and polyphenols with anti•inflammatory effects.
• Turmeric • Contains the active compound curcumin, which has potent anti•inflammatory properties.
• Black pepper • Contains piperine, which has been shown to enhance the bioavailability of curcumin and other anti•inflammatory compounds.

These baked plantain chips make a delicious and healthy snack or side dish that supports an anti•inflammatory diet. The combination of the crispy texture and the earthy, slightly sweet flavor of the plantains, along with the anti•inflammatory spices, creates a tasty and nutritious treat.

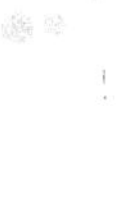

What are the critical points in the recipe (e.g., temperature control, timing)?

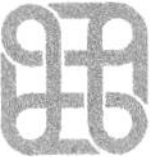 What is the total cooking time, including prep time?

Prep Time : _________________

Cook Time : _________________

Servings : _________________

 Ingredients:

• 1 lb mizuna greens, washed and trimmed
• 2 tbsp olive oil
• 3 cloves garlic, minced
• 1/2 tsp salt
• 1/4 tsp red pepper flakes (optional)

1. Fill a large pot with 1•2 inches of water and bring it to a boil.

2. Place the mizuna greens in a steamer basket and steam for 3•5 minutes, or until the greens are tender.

3. In a small skillet, heat the olive oil over medium heat. Add the minced garlic and sauté for 1•2 minutes, until fragrant.

4. Transfer the steamed mizuna to a serving bowl. Drizzle the garlic•infused olive oil over the greens and toss to coat.

5. Season the steamed mizuna with salt and red pepper flakes (if using).

6. Serve the steamed mizuna with garlic warm.

The mizuna greens provide a delicate, slightly peppery flavor that pairs beautifully with the aromatic garlic. The olive oil helps to coat and lightly dress the greens, while the salt and optional red pepper flakes add depth of flavor.

Mizuna is a nutrient•dense green that is rich in vitamins, minerals, and antioxidants. The garlic also provides anti•inflammatory benefits, making this a great side dish to support overall health.

This simple steamed mizuna with garlic makes a wonderful accompaniment to grilled or roasted proteins, or can be enjoyed on its own as a healthy vegetable side dish.

Is the recipe easy to follow?

112. Steamed mizuna with garlic

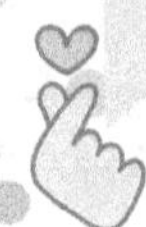

What are the critical points in the recipe (e.g., temperature control, timing)?

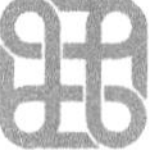
What is the total cooking time, including prep time?

Prep Time : _______________

Cook Time : _______________

Servings   : _______________

Ingredients:

- 2 chayote squash, halved and seeded
- 2 tbsp olive oil
- 1 tsp ground turmeric
- 1/2 tsp salt
- 1/4 tsp black pepper

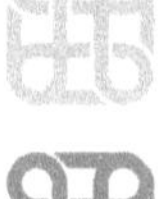
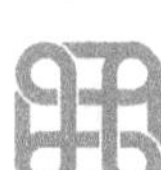
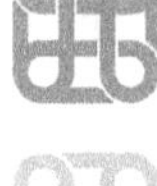
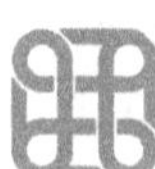
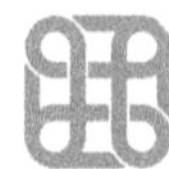

Is the recipe easy to follow?

113. Grilled daikon radish

1. Preheat your oven to 400°F (200°C). Line a baking sheet with parchment paper.

2. Cut the chayote squash in half lengthwise and scoop out the seeds.

3. In a small bowl, mix together the olive oil, turmeric, salt, and black pepper.

4. Brush or drizzle the seasoning mixture over the cut sides of the chayote squash halves, making sure to coat them evenly.

5. Place the seasoned chayote squash halves cut·side up on the prepared baking sheet.

6. Bake for 25·30 minutes, or until the chayote is tender and lightly browned on the edges.

7. Remove the baked chayote squash from the oven and let it cool slightly before serving.

The key anti·inflammatory ingredients in this recipe are:

- Chayote squash · Contains antioxidants and anti·inflammatory compounds like vitamin C and quercetin.
- Olive oil · Rich in monounsaturated fats and polyphenols with anti·inflammatory effects.
- Turmeric · Contains the active compound curcumin, which has potent anti·inflammatory properties.
- Black pepper · Contains piperine, which has been shown to enhance the bioavailability of curcumin and other anti·inflammatory compounds.

What is the total cooking time, including prep time?

Prep Time : _______________

Cook Time : _______________

Servings   : _______________

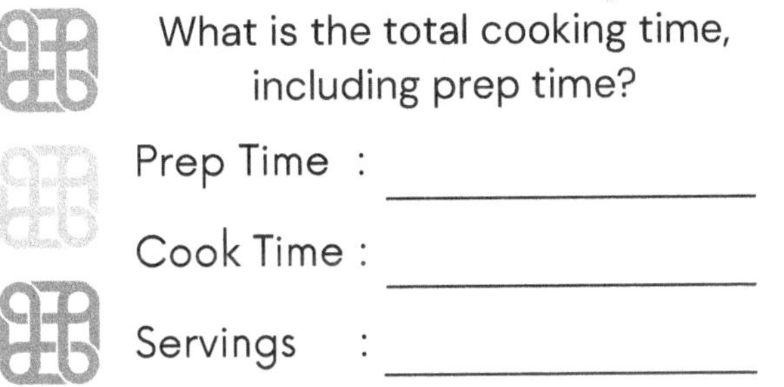

Ingredients:

- 2 chayote squash, halved and seeded
- 2 tbsp olive oil
- 1 tsp ground turmeric
- 1/2 tsp salt
- 1/4 tsp black pepper

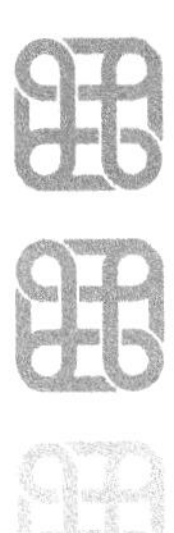

Is the recipe easy to follow?

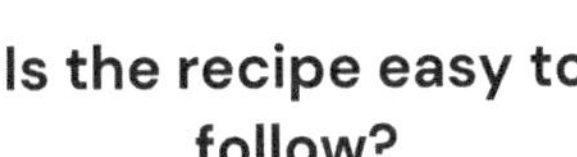
114. Baked chayote squash

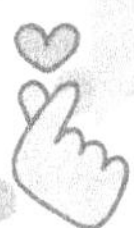

Procedure:

1. Preheat your oven to 400°F (200°C). Line a baking sheet with parchment paper.

2. Cut the chayote squash in half lengthwise and scoop out the seeds.

3. In a small bowl, mix together the olive oil, turmeric, salt, and black pepper.

4. Brush or drizzle the seasoning mixture over the cut sides of the chayote squash halves, making sure to coat them evenly.

5. Place the seasoned chayote squash halves cut•side up on the prepared baking sheet.

6. Bake for 25•30 minutes, or until the chayote is tender and lightly browned on the edges.

7. Remove the baked chayote squash from the oven and let it cool slightly before serving.

The key anti•inflammatory ingredients in this recipe are:

- Chayote squash • Contains antioxidants and anti•inflammatory compounds like vitamin C and quercetin.
- Olive oil • Rich in monounsaturated fats and polyphenols with anti•inflammatory effects.
- Turmeric • Contains the active compound curcumin, which has potent anti•inflammatory properties.
- Black pepper • Contains piperine, which has been shown to enhance the bioavailability of curcumin and other anti•inflammatory compounds.

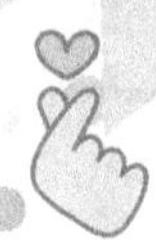

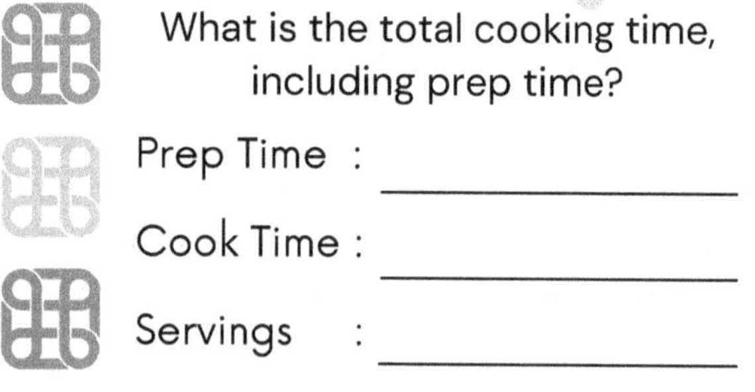

What is the total cooking time, including prep time?

Prep Time : _______________

Cook Time : _______________

Servings : _______________

Ingredients:

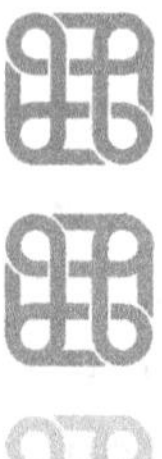
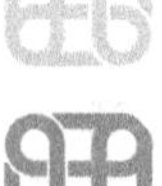
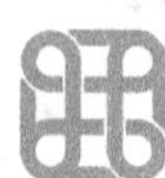

• 1 lb kohlrabi, peeled and cut into 1•inch cubes
• 2 tbsp olive oil
• 1 tsp ground cumin
• 1/2 tsp salt
• 1/4 tsp black pepper

Is the recipe easy to follow?

115. Roasted kohlrabi with cumin

1. Preheat your oven to 400°F (200°C). Line a baking sheet with parchment paper.

2. In a large bowl, toss the kohlrabi cubes with the olive oil, ground cumin, salt, and black pepper until the kohlrabi is evenly coated.

3. Spread the seasoned kohlrabi cubes in a single layer on the prepared baking sheet.

4. Roast the kohlrabi for 25•30 minutes, flipping halfway through, until it is tender and lightly browned.

5. Remove the roasted kohlrabi from the oven and transfer it to a serving dish.

The key anti•inflammatory ingredients in this recipe are:

• Kohlrabi • Contains glucosinolates, vitamin C, and other compounds with anti•inflammatory properties.
• Olive oil • Rich in monounsaturated fats and polyphenols with anti•inflammatory effects.
• Cumin • Contains compounds like cuminaldehyde that have been shown to have anti•inflammatory benefits.
• Black pepper • Contains piperine, which has been demonstrated to have anti•inflammatory effects.

This simple roasted kohlrabi dish makes a great side for an anti•inflammatory diet. The combination of the earthy, slightly sweet kohlrabi with the warm spices of cumin and black pepper creates a delicious and healthy vegetable side.

Enjoy the roasted kohlrabi as a standalone dish or pair it with grilled meats, fish, or other anti•inflammatory•friendly meals.

Thank you for exploring the ***"Anti-Inflammatory 5-Ingredient Cookbook: 5-Ingredient Recipes to Naturally Reduce Inflammation and Enhance Wellness."*** We hope this collection of simple, delicious recipes has inspired you to embrace the power of anti-inflammatory foods and incorporate them into your daily life with ease.

Embracing Simplicity

Throughout this cookbook, we've demonstrated that healthy, anti-inflammatory eating doesn't need to be complicated or time-consuming. By using just five ingredients, you can create flavorful and nutritious meals that support your health and well-being. We've shown that simplicity in cooking can lead to delicious and effective results.

Achieving Wellness

By focusing on anti-inflammatory ingredients, you've taken a significant step towards improving your overall health. Whether you're aiming to reduce chronic inflammation, manage a health condition, or simply feel better day-to-day, the recipes and tips provided in this cookbook offer a practical and enjoyable path to wellness.

Continuing Your Journey

As you continue your journey towards better health, remember that the principles you've learned here can be applied to countless other recipes and cooking techniques. Experiment with new ingredients, try different combinations, and don't be afraid to make these recipes your own. The key is to keep it simple, nutritious, and delicious.

Celebrating Health

Cooking and eating should be enjoyable experiences that bring you closer to your health goals. We hope that the "Anti-Inflammatory 5-Ingredient Cookbook" has helped you discover new favorite meals and a deeper appreciation for the benefits of anti-inflammatory foods.

Thank You

Thank you for choosing this cookbook and taking the time to invest in your health. We hope that the recipes and knowledge shared here will continue to benefit you and your loved ones for years to come. Here's to a life filled with delicious meals, reduced inflammation, and enhanced wellness.

Happy cooking and good health!
Warm regards,